Hammerhead 84

a memoir of persistence

Hammerhead 84

a memoir of persistence

Brett Hartman

Graphite Press

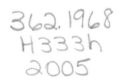

PUBLISHED BY GRAPHITE PRESS

Copyright © 2005 by Brett Hartman

www.graphitepress.com

ISBN-13: 978-0-9755810-0-1
ISBN-10: 0-9755810-0-7

LIBRARY OF CONGRESS CATALOGING-IN-PUBLICATION DATA

Hartman, Brett, 1964–
Hammerhead 84 : a memoir of persistence / Brett Hartman.— 1st ed.
p. cm.
1. Hartman, Brett, 1964—Mental health.
2. Psychoses—Patients—United States—Biography.
3. Psychiatric hospital patients—United States—Biography.
4. Psychoses—Chemotherapy. I. Title.
RC512.H27 2005
362.196'89'0092—dc22

2005008206

PRINTED IN THE UNITED STATES OF AMERICA

First Edition

10 9 8 7 6 5 4 3 2 1

If all you have is a hammer, everything looks like a nail.

Bernard Baruch

Prologue

I MAGINE for a moment that the world you know as real suddenly shifts into a different plane of reality. The rock-solid substance of your former life seems like a mirage—or maybe this new reality is the mirage? You really don't know. It's a scary proposition and invigorating at the same time, certainly not boring. But problems arise when you realize that people around you don't appear to embrace your transformation. In fact, they seem threatened by it, and they're ready to do whatever they can to change you back to the way you were before.

Soon an armed rebellion charges forward to thrust out your new state of being. You fight against this force, but your captors are strong and they have powerful instruments to gain your compliance, forcing you to shift strategy. This struggle goes on for some time and it takes a heavy toll. Every plea you make, every counter-argument is squashed with greater and greater force. In time, you realize that the only strategy left is to save the remaining scattered strands of your life.

This is my story, much like the story of millions of other

people through the years who've found themselves in similar circumstances and battled the same forces. Their journeys are rarely told because the voices that would tell them have been hushed into oblivion. Or, if they do speak out, they become robbed of credibility, relegated to the waste pile of humanity, screaming into a vacuum. Usually they're too numb to realize they have the ability to scream at all.

I tell my story in these pages to add my voice to the many, hoping that mine will not be a muted scream, but a call to greater understanding and perhaps in time to action. Beyond a recounting of my struggle with the mental health system, this memoir is about choices, both good and bad, and their consequences. It's also a tribute to the transformative power of relationships. And, finally, this is a chronicle of persistence—the mysterious will to keep pecking away, often blindly with a naïve kind of stupidity, but forever hopeful that tomorrow will be a better day.

1

Iᴛ's Wednesday the 18ᵗʰ of May 1983, and it's the last day I'll ever have to set foot on the campus of Cardinal Gibbons High. We in the senior class have our final afternoon off, to spend as we like, and we don't have to wear the lousy uniform with the CG logo on every male chest. We're supposed to be adults now with new freedoms. The first of these is to dress as we want.

It's easy to get caught up in the excitement of the day. Four years of the endurance test known as Catholic high school and I'm moving on at last. There'll be no more Sister Hop-a-long, with one leg four inches shorter than the other, lunging around the classroom, taking American History to the outer limits of boredom. No more alcohol-breath Father Lenny, patting me on the ass when he walks by on campus. And, most gratefully, there'll be no more religion class with Mr. Burke and his intolerant drone.

I admit there were good moments in school, like Sister Janet's literature class, which transported me to Ancient Greece. For a semester I lived with Plato and Socrates and the fantastic world of mythology. There was Mr. Baldwin too—disc jockey by night at the Village Zoo and master of Renaissance England by day. Here was my model of the knowledgeable cool. And the parties were another high point, with cold beer in abundance and always a variety of pretty girls to dream about. These were fine moments, but they pale compared to the bright future ahead. My dreams now are of college and the limitless possibilities beyond.

The image I have of college is a bit skewed growing up in Fort Lauderdale, spring break Mecca, where sloppy intoxication is a way of life. It's only fitting that on our last day of high school my classmates and I rise to the stature of model college students by drinking to the outer limits.

First there's a beach party where we drench ourselves in the surf. An hour or so later we're drinking poolside at the home of one of the wealthier students. His backyard patio is stocked with burgers and dogs for the built-in grill and a row of colorful coolers filled with beer. The talk is about college plans and promises to stay in touch.

By late afternoon the celebration loses steam. A group of us wants to go to another party, just off Las Olas Boulevard. I'm pretty well shit-faced by now, so I get my friend Danny to drive. Although I doubt he's any less drunk, I don't ask him to do a sobriety test or anything like that. I just get in the front seat and assume he's okay. Another classmate, Peter, sits corpse-like in the back seat.

We head south on Bayview Drive past our high school and alongside the Coral Ridge Country Club. As we near Oakland Park Boulevard, Danny and I talk about some of the girls in our class. It's an ongoing dialogue whenever we're together, mostly about female body parts. Like Carol and her spectacular ass in the bikini at the party, and why'd she wait four years to put that on display? Or Andrea and her magnificent breasts, which seem too big for the mere word *breasts*. There ought to be another word when they get up to that size. And about Linda—prettiest face on campus—the kind of face that turns guys like me into bumbling idiots.

The conversation fades as we turn left from Sunrise Boulevard onto 20th Street. We pass a series of stucco-clad homes built just after World War II, which makes them some of the oldest structures in town. Danny starts weaving the car back and forth in the lane, speeding through the curves. Maybe he's too messed up to drive. But when I look over at him, he appears to be a man in control, playing the fool for effect.

I've known Danny pretty well through high school, and I like his easygoing attitude. One advantage of being with him is the scarcity of parental presence at his house. We could do almost anything, short of burn the place down, without fear of consequence. And Danny doesn't bother much with consequences. At least that's the sense I get when we're together.

A few months ago we ate at an all-night diner where, after loading up on food and coffee, Danny said we should do a *dine and dash*. For a moment I thought about the morals of food theft and the risk of getting caught, but Danny made it seem like an honorable thing, like a test of courage. So that's what we did, laughing as we sped from the parking lot.

Then there was the time we carved out a hole in an old hardcover science book for the purpose of stealing hamburgers in the cafeteria. It worked as planned. I walked amid the crowded lunch line armed with the book and, at the critical moment, snuck a silver-wrapped hamburger into the enclosure and then paid only for a small Coke. On Fridays we stole fish sandwiches, which required more effort to squeeze into the hole. Once I made the circuit, Danny did likewise, then passed the book around to other select students. No one in a position of authority recognized the grease-laden book making its rounds three or four times a day. We tallied it up, and after about four months use we had racked up over 150 hits.

I wondered how the school was able to square up profits versus inventory, and I was afraid of getting caught, but not enough for me to toss the book. At times I thought Danny was a bad influence on me, leading me down a delinquent path. But that's not the whole story. Neither one of us is likely to win any good citizenship awards.

The road straightens as we approach Victoria Park. We're following a car that's moving as fast as a slug. Danny starts swerving back and forth again, looking for a chance to pass. Then he notices a woman riding along the right side of the road on a 10-speed bicycle. I see her too—a stocky woman dressed in tight orange shorts. My slow brain doesn't register much of an opinion of her one way or the other. But Danny has an idea. He says I ought to reach my hand out the window and slap the woman on her ass. Without thinking the matter through, I prepare to do as he says by reaching out with my right hand cupped.

The only problem is our car. It's still weaving back and forth and I can't judge where my hand will land. I'm afraid we'll hit the woman with the front bumper, so I begin to pull back.

But it's too late. My elbow strikes the woman's buttock hard, knocking her off the bike. The feeling of pressure on my arm is followed by a clanging sound of metal smacking pavement. I turn around and see that the woman isn't moving. Danny notices the car in front of us pulling over. The driver must have seen the whole thing, so our impulse to flee the scene is overruled.

Once parked, Danny, Peter and I bolt out of the car and assume the new role of helpful roadside assistants. I can't say much of anything, and my brain is a mess. If I say what I'm thinking it would be something like, "Jesus, shit, what did I do? Holy fucking mother of shit, what did I do? Holy shit, Jesus, No!"

But instead, I'm silent except for the sound of my chest pounding like a drum. I stand by the unconscious woman as blood trickles from the top of her head and face. She doesn't move, and she looks as good as dead, except for the hopeful sign that she's breathing. That's the only good thing.

In a matter of seconds a crowd is attracted. Neighbors congregate around the woman and her bike. Then two police cars pull onto the grass to make room for an ambulance, which arrives a few minutes later and blocks a lane of traffic.

With paramedics, traffic cops and detectives all on alert mode, it's an unreal scene. Even though I've been drinking all afternoon, I couldn't be more sober now. It seems the same is true of Danny, who looks like the picture of calm when a detective comes over to question us. My words are too pressurized right now—sure to give me away—so I step back and let Danny do the talking. The detective already questioned the woman driving in front of us, who must have given full account of our misdeeds. But Danny tells a different version of the story. He says the woman on the bike was riding too far out on the street, requiring us to swerve in order to miss her, but unfortunately we clipped her anyway. Looking down the street I see no bicycle lane, so the story seems to have credibility.

Impressed by Danny's performance, I try to pull myself together. I add my own twisted take on reality, hoping the heart palpitations won't give me away. I tell the detective that my arm was propped out of the window as a style of sitting in a relaxed manner, as if that's how I always sit in a car.

It's hard hearing the lie as I'm telling it, besides the fact that it sounds too stupid, even for me. The cop writes down my story, but I figure he can see right through it. I picture Danny and me riding to the Broward County Jail, handcuffs and all.

Amazingly, the cop lets us go. He tells us to forget about going to the party, to drive straight home and to know that he'll be getting in touch with us. Meanwhile, the woman lying on the street is taken away in the ambulance with no word of her prognosis. I would learn later that her name is Lois.

The drive home is a miserable affair. My brain races from one awful scenario to another, and it doesn't help to see Danny looking so calm. He says he's confident that our story will stick. I don't know what to think. After debating our strategy, we're quiet for the rest of the drive. In the backseat, Peter looks like a punitive father who knows we'll pay for our sins. I can feel his judgment.

I'm starting to hate Danny for getting me into this mess, and I hate myself for being so stupid and suggestible. How could I have been such a dumb-ass? The only excuses are drunkenness and the excitement of the day. Neither is good enough. I feel like one of those scumbags you read about in the newspaper—the kind you feel good about when they're locked away for years. Like the scumbag, the last thing I want to do is admit my guilt and pay the legal consequences. It's not an option. I've got plans for the future. I'm set to enroll at Auburn University in the fall. After that, I'll have a successful career, get married, have kids, build a house and live out my years in suburban bliss. Hard time in the Florida prison system isn't part of the plan.

I feel a small measure of relief upon arriving home. I want to hibernate here awhile. I can hang out with my sisters and my mother and pretend the dreaded thing never happened. My classmates are sure to party through the night without a single care, but I don't want to see any of them. Maybe they'd draw me into committing yet another unforgivable act.

Sitting at the kitchen table, I eat almost nothing for dinner and say even less. My mother asks about my day and about the excitement of finishing high school. I say vague and pleasant things. After dinner I transfer myself to the couch and watch something mindless on TV. But I can't focus on the show or the conversation between my mother and sisters.

Once the dishes are done, the phone rings. My mother answers. The man on the other end identifies himself as a detective with the Fort Lauderdale Police Department. Then he gives my mother an account of the incident during which she looks over at me on the couch.

I'm trying to appear calm, gazing at a *M*A*S*H* rerun, but I can't help noticing the look of stress on my mother's face. Then I hear her say, "He's sitting right here. Do you want to talk to him?"

The detective must have said no because my mother doesn't hand me the phone, which relieves me beyond measure. But my overall fear grows. I've always thought of my home as a safe haven, removed from the dangers of the outside world. One phone call from a cop is enough to change that. No longer aware of the television, I drop my head and cover my face with my hands. I'm the picture of shame.

My mother tells the detective that he can count on our cooperation. After some stiff pleasantries, the call is over. Then she looks at me with a hard stare. She wants an explanation.

I tell her how it happened, mostly as Danny and I explained to the detective. It's a monumental struggle getting the words out, but by the end of the story I think she believes me and she'll help in any way she can. She says she's always distrusted Danny and thinks of him as a bad kid. Here we find common ground for the moment. Danny's an easy scapegoat.

The next day I tell my father about the incident. He also lives in Fort Lauderdale, about two miles from us, having divorced my mother back in 1971. When I tell him I have something to say, I can't look him in the eye and I give him a watered down version, again with Danny the main culprit.

My dad listens without interrupting. When I'm finished, he tells me that it's not so bad and that everything will turn out okay. Then he talks about the legal aspects of the situation and what I should do to defend myself. And so Lois, the woman I nearly killed, becomes Lois the legal adversary. My dad and I have successfully managed to smooth the whole thing over. I'm relieved that he isn't upset with me, but I still have the cold sense of getting away with something rotten. I know this isn't in the same category as dodging the bill at a diner or pilfering hamburgers in a school lunch line. Sooner or later I'll pay for this one. My hope is for later—much later.

Our graduation ceremony is held at Parker Playhouse, near Fort Lauderdale's central business district. Nearly 300 of us are dressed in red caps and gowns. Faculty, clergy, friends and family are all here, mostly dressed in formal wear. The smart ones are wearing shorts, owing to the sticky heat of the day. My mother, my two sisters and maternal grandparents are here. Even a few of my mother's friends from the church choir have come to show their support.

Notably absent is my father, who delivers a baby instead of coming to the ceremony. He's an obstetrician in private practice, and he's on call around the clock. In this case, delivering a baby instead of coming to my graduation is a convenient thing because my father is never eager to spend time with my mother or her parents. There's still bitterness over the divorce coming from both sides, and there's the simple fact that my parents don't like each other. To show that he feels bad about not coming to the ceremony he gave me $500, which is the amount he'd have to shell out for another doctor to cover for him. I can't say whether the money is worth his absence.

After the ceremony, I pull together a small party at my house with six fellow graduates. There's to be no driving around drunk and no women on 10-speed bicycles—just a bunch of guys drinking beer and eating deli sandwiches. When the beer runs out, we arrange for someone to get us more. We make a pyramid on the kitchen table with all the empty cans, leaving little room for anything else.

Soon we're drunk and hot, looking for a way to refresh ourselves. Normally we'd plunge into the swimming pool, beer cans in hand. It's a fact that any self-respecting South Floridian with a decent income has a functioning pool. But unfortunately, my mother and her friends from the choir are occupying ours, wading around, talking shop about church politics and the choir scene. Being in the water with them would no doubt kill our buzz.

With the pool off limits, we're left with the undesirable alternative of swimming in the canal behind the back yard. There's a 30-foot motorboat docked back there, owned by a man my mother knows from choir. He rarely uses the thing and cleans it even less. Still, I don't think he'd appreciate a bunch of drunken teenagers traipsing over his boat, jumping off its side. But he isn't here to complain.

Canals in Fort Lauderdale are a brackish, brown color with a petroleum film on much of the surface. They have an appearance not unlike the inside of a toilet after you've had a bad bowl of conch chowder. The only fish you can catch in the canals are catfish, blowfish and mullet, but the mullet are either too smart or too lazy for bait, so you have to catch them with a snag hook. Regardless of what you catch, none of it is edible. At least I never hear of people eating things out of the canal and then living to tell about it.

There's a degree of danger in taking a canal plunge, which has nothing to do with the fish. It's the barnacles covering all stationary objects that you need to avoid. These crustaceans are sharp enough to break skin and are said to be breeding grounds for all sorts of bacterial stuff you don't want in your system. My mother warns about the risk of catching hepatitis, and she tells us how ridiculous we are. "Look around," she says, "do you see anyone else swimming there?"

I don't know about the risk of hepatitis, but she's right

about the lack of canal bathers. Still her words have no effect.

So here we are, high school graduates, drunk and laughing and splashing around in the canal, trying to keep our extremities clear of the dreaded barnacles. It's mindless fun and it helps ward off the terrible thoughts in my brain.

Just below the surface is my fear over Lois and the legal authorities clamping down on me. The thought arises that there may be two people struggling inside me—one who carries on as if everything is cool, like a regular guy, and a second person emerging who fears that it could all crack in an instant.

2

T HE summer of 1983 isn't likely to make it as a monumental time in history. Newsworthy events are mostly a blur, hardly registering a flicker of importance in my little world. And yet this is my time. It's the beginning of a new era for me.

Among world events, there's an ongoing struggle between us and the Soviets, who continue to spy on us while meddling in Afghanistan's civil war, bombing out that country's infrastructure. The U.S. Congress argues over a new proposal to build space-based weapons of mass destruction, adding new tension to the Cold War. As always since the late 1940's, there are clashes between the Palestinians and Israelis over territorial rights. Worldwide drought with subsequent famine and starvation plague much of the Third World, especially the midsection of Africa. Pictures of skeletal Ethiopian children serve as a jarring emblem of world hunger.

Americans are mildly concerned about our security in the aftermath of the U.S. Embassy bombing in Beirut, but we're more concerned about the mounting federal deficit, which has doubled over the past 12 months. Congress blames President Reagan, and Reagan blames Congress. We side with Reagan, as his approval ratings reach their highest level since his inauguration in 1981.

The economy is humming along after some sluggish years, recording new highs on Wall Street. IBM is the envy of the business world with its PC, and Diet Coke is the new beverage of choice. The car people want is the Porsche 928, yet the one they buy is the Ford Tempo.

We're listening to the music of David Bowie, Men at Work, the Stray Cats, Michael Jackson and the Police. We're packing theatres to see *Star Wars III: Return of the Jedi*, *Flashdance* and *Trading Places*. In sports, the USFL completes their first and nearly last season. Turn on the TV and you might witness the stardom of Mr. T on the hit show *A-Team*, which tells you how sophisticated we are as a country. Other popular shows include *Magnum PI*, *Hart to Hart*, *Facts of Life* and *Fantasy Island*.

We fly two politically correct space shuttle missions during the summer. The first flight includes the first female astronaut, while the second features the first black astronaut. Locally, in Miami's Biscayne Bay, the conceptual artist Christo recently completed wrapping 11 islands in pink polypropylene at a cost of $3.2 million.

I work for Van Arsdale's furniture moving company throughout the summer as I've done the previous two. The job is exhausting, especially in the drenching humidity of a South Florida summer. By 10 A.M. my shirt is saturated and by noon I stink. The other men smell just as bad, which is especially noxious on the drive back to the warehouse after a full house move. The person in the middle suffers the most.

Tony is the easiest of the bunch to get along with. He's an Italian from Westchester County who likes to brag about his exploits in New York City. The way he tells it, you'd think Manhattan is a fantasyland with an endless entourage of sex-starved women. Tony builds up a certain momentum when he's talking, and he doesn't like it when someone interrupts for details, such as to ask how much he paid for his encounters.

With all his praise of New York, I wonder why he lives in Fort Lauderdale, but I know he's prone to exaggeration. Like whenever our moving van passes by an attractive woman, Tony carries on like a sex-crazed freak. He honks the horn, waves and says strange things like, "Give me some honey!" Then he drives on, talking about how *hot* she was for the next five miles. It's like he was just released from prison and hasn't seen a pretty female in years.

Tony's behind-the-wheel antics take a sinister shift when another driver does something stupid. I shrink down in my seat, trying to hide while Tony blasts the other driver with the full armament of horn-honking, middle finger shaking and shouts of "asshole" and "dumb-fuck!" The surprising thing is his driving, flawless throughout the episode.

Worse for me are the times when we pass a woman riding her bicycle alongside the truck. My reaction is almost reflexive. Body turns to plywood while I make sure to keep my hands, arms and elbows firmly inside the cabin of the truck. Whatever I was thinking before is gone. All I can do is replay the horror of Lois and her 10-speed bike.

Tony and the other men aren't aware of my change in posture, and they don't know anything about the event that consumes my brain. No one at Van Arsdale's knows about it, and that's how I want it.

Near the end of July, Tony gets assigned to drive the big rig on a statewide move, which includes drop-offs in Daytona Beach, Jacksonville and Tallahassee. I'm honored when he chooses me as his coworker on the trip. Most of our business is local, so this is a special privilege—to get paid while driving and sleeping in motels. I think of how great it'll be to escape for a while and earn extra cash along the way.

Without a chauffeur's license I can't drive the truck, but Tony says it's my duty to keep him awake and alert throughout the trip. This is no task at all because the man is nearly always wired like a chicken coop and probably even more when he's out on the open road. He rattles on about his past, and he's never boring but almost always crude. He isn't mean though, and I like the flow of talk when we're sitting in the cabin of the truck. It's when we're in earshot of other human beings that he turns into an embarrassment.

Sitting in the truck cruising through the miles, I find it easier to relax. It's a time when the concerns of the outside world have less impact. For a while I can almost forget about the $1.2 million lawsuit that Lois brought against Danny and me. It staggers my brain to imagine paying even a fraction of that. In the truck, I can put aside the fear of being sent away to prison or the concern that my father will have to shell out a fortune in legal expenses to keep me out. And sitting here miles from home, it's easier to ignore the stream of letters and phone messages from lawyers. It's a short break from the jolting fear of what might happen.

During the rare moments of silence, I think about leaving Fort Lauderdale and starting a new life at Auburn. When I get there I think I'll major in criminology—it might come in handy someday.

Back in the fall of '82, I took on the task of choosing a good college and figuring out where I could get accepted. My grades were mediocre, as were my test scores, so I wasn't in the running for slots at the more prestigious schools. By playing football, my stock could have risen. This option sounded fine for a time, especially when the mailbox filled with letters and flashy brochures from football programs across the country. I got calls from coaches at the University of Miami and Florida State, and letters from as far away as Brown and the University of Texas at El Paso.

All the attention was flattering, but by the end of the football season I decided not to play at the college level. I made that decision the night Cardinal Gibbons played Ely High. As the biggest offensive lineman on the team, it was my job to block Victor Morris, who was by all accounts the strength of the Ely defense. He was a huge black defensive end said to be solid muscle, and he had a quickness that was uncanny. The entire week leading up to the game I was bombarded with warnings and advice on how to contain this super human force. As we approached kick-off, with the sight of him warming up with his team, I unintentionally placed Victor among the elite forces of the universe. He could've been the reincarnation of Achilles, ready to slay everyone in sight, filling the Intracoastal Waterway with the blood of all South Floridians not associated with Ely High School.

And my fear was warranted. I was beaten badly on nearly every play, and we had to resort to double-teaming him most of the game. One play late in the third quarter epitomized the game for me. It was a pass play where I had to block Victor on the left side of the line. Once the ball was snapped, I charged into his chest and actually felt him moving backward. It was almost unbelievable, and I was overjoyed—that is, until I realized Victor was backing up on purpose to intercept a pass, which he did. Then, with little effort, he was able to swat me aside like a rag doll and coast into the end zone. That's when I knew I wouldn't be extending my football career beyond high school.

So I turned to the larger state schools, which are more affordable and have fairly easy acceptance standards. I wanted to get out of South Florida, maybe even the whole state, but I had no idea beyond that. When my closest friend Phil said he might be going to Auburn, in Alabama, there was something about it that felt right.

Then, after Phil and I took a road trip there in the winter of '83, the decision was all but made. We liked the red brick architecture and the orderliness of the campus, and we were struck by the friendly atmosphere. Our first evening featured a basketball game at the Coliseum during which Auburn defeated Georgia in thrilling fashion. The game was punctuated by two slam dunks, courtesy of Charles Barkley, sending Auburn fans into hysterics. Afterward, we partied alongside college students, taking full notice of the beautiful Southern girls. This trip was more than enough to clinch my four year commitment.

In retrospect, choosing Auburn had more to do with Phil than any other factor, though my pride won't let me admit it. Realizing what a mess I got myself into now, I'm even more grateful to have him nearby.

Phil has been my closest friend since we were both six years old. We live four houses apart from each other in a wealthy neighborhood off Bayview Drive. I remember the first day my family moved into our house in 1970. After exploring the inside, I walked alone down the street about 30 feet when I noticed another boy coming toward me. We stopped and looked at each other, vaguely recognizing the other from kindergarten at Pine Crest. I yelled Phil's name with boyish enthusiasm, and he yelled mine back with equal feeling. From that day forward we've been best friends.

It helps that we've shared a lot of interests along the way, like tree forts, cars and football and eventually the female form. We admired each other's toys, but Phil always came out ahead when it came to material acquisitions. I remember envying him for the bike he had, which was a bright orange Schwinn five-speed with a banana seat, front disc brakes, extended handlebars and working shock absorbers. His dad must have shelled out quite a sum for the thing. Meanwhile, I had a lowly one-speed affair with chipped paint. As if to underscore how pathetic my bike was, we took turns ghost-riding it down the street to see who could push it farthest before it crashed onto someone's front lawn.

After school when it wasn't raining, we played in the front yard of my house. We climbed the sea grape tree, which dominated the landscape, and one of our favorite hobbies was to play with the mulch chips under the big tree. Phil and I spent hours digging a network of miniature dirt roads within the mulch. The windy roads connected boulders and bushes, which figured to be buildings in our minds. Our hands and knees and faces got filthy, and there were roaches and lizards to contend with, but none of it mattered. We were absorbed in our creation—a functional town for miniature humans and their Tonka toy vehicles. When complete, we stood back and marveled at the scene below. Then we messed it up to start a new design.

We also tried making original music. We employed my father's discarded reel-to-reel tape deck with an external microphone, which one of us tapped on to serve as a drum beat. I played a total of three chords—the extent of my skill—on my mother's old classical guitar, and Phil and I sang songs in rough harmony. Lyrically, the songs ranged from obscure to morbid, with such titles as *I Love to Carry Fertilizer up the Hills of Montezuma*, *The Black Dog Crapped on the Fence*, *Little Baby Duckies Grinding in the Gears of a Semi* and, our favorite, *Razor Blades*. It was hard getting through the songs without cracking up, and we were smart enough to realize that we had zero musical talent.

Phil and I had our share of fights as well, which were pretty much limited to verbal assaults. The outcome of these followed a predictable pattern. The two of us pledged mutual hatred for the other, vowing never to see the other again. Then we stormed off in opposite directions after which followed a period of two or three weeks of non-communication. It was like a cold war where we each tried to get information about the other through our perceived allies in the neighborhood.

Finally, after the boredom reached an intolerable level, one of us would break down and visit the other. To me, it was an act of supreme humility—to admit I couldn't outlast Phil and then to admit being wrong. But, in no time at all, it didn't matter who did the making up. As if nothing bad had happened, we were best friends again.

Over the years Phil and I marked some important milestones together. At age 12, we were sitting in his family room when the phone rang. It was someone from the Imperial Point Medical Center informing him that his mother had just died of lung cancer. I remember trying to console Phil, but all I could do was cry.

When Phil and I were nine, we had matching red bathing suits with a fish pattern. At 15, we had matching red motorcycles, his with a fancy luggage rack. In that same year, while on a boat trip in Key Largo, the two of us got badly intoxicated for the first time. That summer we lobbied our parents to attend the local Catholic high school, even though neither of us is Catholic. And we both joined the freshman football team.

The coach spotted early on that Phil and I were a nearly inseparable pair. He sought to exploit this during a fully-uniformed hitting drill by making us square off against each other. Neither of us wanted to comply. So, when the whistle blew, we plowed into each other with all the force of a wet sponge. This wasn't what the coach was looking for. So he had us hit each other again and then again, until the crack of our pads could be heard throughout the practice field.

I raised my left hand to call it off but instead caught the tip of my thumb in Phil's face mask. The thumb twisted at a bad angle as Phil pulled his head away. It hurt like a bitch, and then

I noticed the nail turning all purple. The next six months were a constant reminder of the incident as a new thumbnail grew in to replace the old.

In our freshman year of high school, Phil started complaining about shortness of breath, and he was coughing all over the place. Soon his doctor diagnosed Hodgkin's disease. Phil underwent chemotherapy and later, radiation treatments. About a month into treatment his condition took a bad turn, which forced his admission into Imperial Point Medical Center—a place not known for cheery outcomes.

I visited him after football practice and tried to keep the conversation positive, but I couldn't help noticing him looking more and more grim. Before all this started, he was overweight and full of energy. But now he was tired, balding and thin as a rail with shingles on his arms. Still he kept his spirits up, even on the day he was fitted for a wig.

The most disturbing image for me was the look on the face of Phil's father. After seeing Phil one evening in a semiconscious state, I boarded the elevator along with his father and stepmother. I stood across from Phil's dad, having always feared the man, and I looked sideways at him. His new wife stood a few feet away. I caught a glimpse of him struggling to hold back tears, but they came anyway. He said maybe Phil would get better, but he didn't sound very convincing about it.

I went home and cried hard that evening and did something I never do. I prayed to God to save Phil's life. I've never been a strong believer in the power of prayer, and I doubt my feeble message had any effect. But after a few months Phil mounted a recovery. One of the respiratory therapists called it a miraculous recovery. I remember the day he returned to school—minus 30 pounds and sporting a clumsy hairpiece—with a kind of brave determination that was foreign to me. I was happy and also scared for him.

Gradually, Phil returned to his old self. He even returned to the football team in his junior year. But even now, as we prepare to go off to college, his hair has yet to make a full comeback. Small price to pay, I guess.

3

B Y the end of August, I'm preparing for the trip from Fort Lauderdale to Auburn. It's the journey I've longed for since the beginning of summer. I shop for clothes with my mother, who wants to equip me for all types of weather related phenomena. It's as if I'm traveling to Alaska for an adventure in the Klondike. But my frame of reference has always been South Florida, where any place north of Jacksonville represents *The North* and the possibility of snow. I don't think I've ever owned a pair of winter gloves or a hat, and I wonder whether such accessories will be needed at all.

After shopping, I find my mother rummaging through my belongings with a black felt-tipped pen, applying my initials on every garment in a supposedly inconspicuous spot. She will not be held responsible for any lost or stolen items.

The car I drive is a 1977 two-toned, brown and tan, Chevy El Camino. With its big V8 and four barrel carburetor it's like an angry animal, tires spinning on command, and I'm proud of the work I've done to it. This includes installing a heart thumping sound system and a wooden deck on the back platform.

As the trip to Auburn approaches I'm filled with a new fear, which is that I won't be allowed to go at all, or at least not until my legal problems are resolved. This could take a year or more, and I'm still worried about being sent away to jail. I won't find out for several months that Lois actually dropped the criminal charges against Danny and me. This was merciful beyond all expectation. But she continues to pursue the civil suit, alleging memory loss and other hardships.

It's a blessing when the judge and the attorneys agree to let me correspond with them from the State of Alabama. My lawyer arranged a deposition to be held when I return to Florida for winter break. That seems a long way off from now. Meanwhile, I hope to put Lois and the whole mess out of my brain. My strategy is to block out all the bad feelings and avoid considering the legal fallout. I think the longer I ignore the situation the less impact it'll have in the future. I keep everything inside, locked away from people who might otherwise try to offer their support.

On a sticky Friday in mid-September, Phil and I pack our respective vehicles for the trip. Classes at Auburn are scheduled on the quarter system in which the academic terms match the four seasons, so we don't start classes until late September. It feels like a big deal to be leaving at last, and my mother turns it into a bigger deal with the long farewell wishes and warnings about being careful. My sisters and our dog Rolex stand by for photos of the big sendoff. I'm happy and sad at the same time, and I feel even sadder when I see my younger sister Julia tearing up. Phil and I need to get out of here before it gets too sappy.

The trip is approximately 650 miles with the longest part of it taking us through the midsection of Florida, via the Turnpike and Interstate 75. This may be the most boring and painfully long stretch of highway in the country. We start along the

Eastern coastline and veer west at Fort Pierce into a sea of orange groves and billboards. We pass through Orlando and then Ocala, stopping for the night in Gainesville to visit friends at the University of Florida.

We spend a night of beer drinking and flirting with freshmen Gator girls. After a hung-over breakfast at Skeeter's Big Biscuit, Phil and I are back on the road, heading north again on I-75. By the time we pass Lake City and emerge into the State of Georgia, we think we've accomplished something big. It's probably a bigger deal for me than it is for Phil. I have a kind of deluded belief that if I manage to get out of Florida my troubles will fade away. It's like equating statehood with state of mind.

We stop for lunch near Valdosta. And then we're off the interstate, speeding through the southwest corner of Georgia on state roads. Phil leads the way with his trusty radar detector.

One notable stopping point is the town of Plains—home to former president Jimmy Carter. It's the kind of town you could drive through at 60 miles an hour and barely register a thought, except to wonder why anyone would want to live here. Carter's house is set back far from the road, hardly visible, blocked by an impressive fence and hedgerow. That would have been the only structure worth seeing, but we do stop at the general store to urinate and pick up some Mountain Dew for the caffeine boost. The store has a wide assortment of items featuring the former president's face, which we don't find hard to resist. The thought of buying a six-pack of Billy Beer comes and goes. Other than the store clerk, Phil and I seem to be the only living humans in town.

Near Columbus, Georgia, I'm able to pick up a faint AM broadcast of the football game featuring Auburn versus the University of Texas. I flash my lights for Phil to pull over so he too can enjoy the game's coverage on his radio. Once we pass the state line into Alabama, things are looking grim for the Auburn Tigers on the gridiron. It's clear that the game is beyond reach. Auburn will suffer its first (and ultimately its only) defeat of the season.

This casts a spell of depression on both of us as we pull up to campus to start our college career.

The mood doesn't improve when I discover where I'll be living for the foreseeable future. The dormitory, Magnolia Hall, is a dilapidated brick structure nearly a hundred years old. It has tiny rooms with inadequate air conditioning and common bathrooms on each floor. Like creatures infesting the dead, we of Magnolia Hall are called *maggots*, and it's an apt description. In two years the building would be demolished, but that would be two years too late.

To make matters worse, my roommate Rob is a nonstop talker with boundless energy, far too much energy to contain in this shoebox of a room. He's from West Palm Beach—a fellow Floridian—and it's my impression that the University sticks us Floridians together with the expectation that our regional bond would translate into a good living arrangement. Nothing could be further from the truth. I'm able to last a total of six days with Rob and Magnolia Hall.

Meanwhile, Phil is living it up in the comparatively plush Caroline Draughon Village Extension, or CDV. Located on the outskirts of campus, these are modern two-bedroom apartments for four students with a large central kitchen and a spacious bathroom. There's even central air conditioning. With likeable roommates who don't display the habit of nonstop chatter, Phil is living on easy street.

For me, the combined effect of Rob, Magnolia Hall and the influx of letters from lawyers is enough to sink me down to a new low. I don't want to admit it, but I'm homesick for the old comforts, like my bedroom, my shower, home-cooked meals and the unquestioning love of my mother. Here at Auburn it's daily heartache, and I can't stop envying Phil who's doing fine in his little college paradise.

Not ready to admit defeat, I take two significant steps to improve my situation. First, I plead with the Housing Authority to find a vacancy at CDV, like it's their duty in the interest of human welfare to give me a break. With persistence, after several days of back and forth, I get a spot left by an early dropout. I need to convince my father to put up extra money for the higher rent. He must sense the desperation in my voice when I tell him how Magnolia Hall feels like a death sentence. Without fuss, my dad agrees to the rent increase.

The second step is to convince Phil to go with me on a weekend road trip back to Fort Lauderdale, which given the distance is totally impractical. But we do it anyway, driving in Phil's brown Celica into the wee hours of the night. On the drive down, Phil admits to being homesick too, so we both make marvelous plans to reconnect with the pattern of life we knew before Auburn.

This turns out to be a fool's errand, as we have time to do little more than wash our dirty clothes. But the trip helps me get a better perspective when I'm back on campus. I'm discovering that I can't go home, despite missing parts of my old home life. Auburn is home now. With this change of view things get a little easier to handle.

A popular way to bridge home life with college is to join a fraternity. It isn't a thing I'd do on my own, but with Phil's persuasiveness and all the free beer you can handle it's a legitimate option. Phil and I visit the string of fraternities lining Magnolia Avenue during rush week. This is the time when all the fraternities try to convince you what a great bunch of guys they are—how they have more cold beer, prettier women, better parties and a better equipped fraternity house than all the others. For some it's a hard sell.

The place we keep returning to is the Alpha Tau Omega

house. Some of the perks here, as with most of the others, are the instant presence of women called *little sisters*, beer parties every week and a group of guys with a relaxed attitude toward life. The ATO fraternity isn't remarkable in any one of these areas, but they seem to have the essentials covered in a balanced sort of way. So by the end of rush week Phil and I agree to become ATO pledges and to go through initiation during the upcoming winter quarter.

Meanwhile at CDV, Phil and I spend a lot of time with our respective roommates. We decided early on that it wasn't a good idea for us to room together, given our propensity for arguments, which might take days to resolve. It's a stubbornness both of us share and it calls for a buffer between us, lest we give up the voice of reason and brutalize each other. Sleeping might be a problem under such conditions.

Phil's roommate Dean, or "Deano" as he prefers to be called, is a likeable guy with a storehouse of knowledge on music and sports. He comes from a tiny redneck town in the southeast corner of Alabama—a place detached from modern society where the local Hardee's may be the cultural high point.

It's laughable when we first hear Deano talk in his thick, low toned Southern accent. Phil and I are sitting at the kitchen table eating pizza when Deano first arrives flanked by his mother and grandmother. He's carrying a laundry basket full of clothes, upon which is perched an unopened bag of Golden Flakes potato chips. His first words are, "Hi y'all, want some Golden Flakes?"

Phil and I give a perfunctory greeting and say no thanks to the chips. Then we look at each other, struggling not to laugh. To us, it's as if we just made contact with the Martians, and they're trying to win us over with potato chips.

Across the lawn from Phil and Deano in the CDV complex is the building where I now reside. My new roommate is a Connecticut native who looks like Moe from *The Three Stooges*. His name is Phil, which isn't a viable option because of the confusion of having two Phils in our midst. Since the latter Phil's last name is Gordon, we give him the nickname Flash, in homage to the comic book superhero.

We could've chosen the nickname Reagan, as it soon becomes clear that Flash is a hard core Republican and devout Reaganite. One of his imperative daily rituals is watching the evening news. Whenever our 40th president is featured, Flash gets transfixed. It's as if every word the President says leaves a golden imprint on Flash's brain. Argue against his merits and you argue against immutable truth. We tease him about his Republican devotions, trying to distract him during Reagan's speeches, but he's not deterred. At one point I say I'll be supporting Jesse Jackson in the upcoming Democratic primary just to see the look on his face.

Flash is an ROTC man who takes very seriously his duty to serve and protect our country. Befitting the military role, he's a fussy dresser and, when there are occasions for him to don his formal officer's attire, he does so with exacting precision and pride. He can't help but smile in his immaculate uniform. By contrast, I usually wear tattered polo shirts un-tucked and the same pair of faded blue jeans each day, washing them on a weekly basis. Flash and I aren't soul mates by any stretch, but we get along pretty well. We can talk for hours about interesting things, which makes it a good match.

In the other bedroom of our apartment reside two engineering students who Flash and I hardly ever see outside the confines of CDV. One of these suitemates, Mark, is also in the military reserves. He's a humorless sort who's tough to get a reaction out of. Even at football games with his girlfriend, he's the picture of stoicism. Flash says that Mark has a nearly perfect grade point average, which I guess is a nice reward for being a killjoy. But I don't think it's worth it.

Our other suitemate, Fred, is even stranger. Here's a morbidly obese hermit who hoards his belongings, even food and cookware, on his side of the bedroom. He rarely leaves the apartment except to go to class or shop for food. Even during home football games he sits in his darkened room, watching the action on a small TV.

Fred's also a penny pincher who buys the generic version of whatever he needs. I can understand living on a fixed income and opting for generic products when the money runs low. But unlike Fred I can't imagine going generic on beer, which is one of the most valuable commodities on the Auburn campus, next to women and football. I look in our refrigerator and see a collection of plain yellow cans with no identifying marks except for the block-lettered printing of the word BEER. Fred gets teased about this, and he's taking it too seriously. Soon he resorts to storing his beer in a cooler at the foot of his bed.

I feel sorry for Fred. It seems like he's hiding dark secrets, but I don't say anything. It's easier to avoid him and let it go. I've got secrets of my own to keep.

The burden of Lois still floods my thoughts, but there's a weekly reprieve. On Saturdays I lapse into the fanaticism of Auburn Football. And the team is worthy of my heroic dreams. One by one, after the Texas loss, Auburn finds a way to win, sometimes in ugly fashion and sometimes through pulverization.

Home games are especially exciting. Jordon-Hare Stadium dominates the landscape, seating over 85,000 people. On game day with a packed stadium, the small town of Auburn becomes the third most populated city in the state.

I'm lucky to attend the school while Bo Jackson graces the gridiron. Here's a man who can break through a defensive front and bolt loose for a touchdown from anywhere on the field. It happens enough to know that it's always a possibility. The crowd watches with expectancy whenever he gets the ball. The chant "Go Bo! Go Bo! Go Bo!" fills the stadium. Defensive teams fear him like no other.

After the game is over, with the Tigers victorious, a throng of fans congregates at the center of town for a traditional celebration. Revelers toss rolls of toilet paper into the air so the entire thing streams out and drapes itself onto the surrounding trees and power lines. The final effect is akin to a Salvador Dali snowstorm.

By far the most important game of the season is the state championship between Auburn and the University of Alabama, known as the Iron Bowl. The game is held in Birmingham, which is supposed to be a neutral site, but it's actually more like a second home for the Crimson Tide.

Late in the fall of '83 Phil and I set off for the game with two female classmates from the Birmingham area. At first it looks as though the game won't even take place with the ominous clouds, the high winds and the threat of tornadoes. But to cancel or even delay a game of this magnitude in the State of Alabama is unthinkable.

It rains hard for most of the afternoon, forcing both teams into a ground struggle. Bo Jackson proves to be the superior ball carrier. He gets a total of 256 yards, including two breakaway touchdown runs of 69 and 71 yards apiece. That last run put Auburn ahead for good. Our side of the stadium goes from party atmosphere into a wild kind of joy. We now have state bragging rights for a year, until we meet again.

Phil and I and our companions stay late after the game with the Auburn faithful, yelling our voices hoarse, chanting and mocking the Bama fans. We're drunk on the rum we smuggled into the stadium, but the real partying has yet to start.

We go to a band party where I stand glazed, half-stupefied, holding a gallon jug of draft beer while leaning against a loudspeaker. Later, we stop at a couple of clubs in downtown Birmingham where Auburn fans have taken over. We talk about the game with unwavering excitement and speculate on who we'll play in the upcoming Sugar Bowl. When we're thoroughly wasted and losing steam, we get a ride back to the home of our friendly hostess.

The house is an extravagant hillside mansion in the suburb of Mountain Brook where you can see the city of Birmingham from a bay window in the living room. A telescope on a tripod is perched by the window to satisfy your voyeuristic side. But we spend the night in the basement recreation room, drinking Evan Williams straight out of the bottle.

At around three in the morning, Phil and I work our way into a besotted argument about the Auburn quarterback—Randy something. Phil makes the point that the player is a lousy excuse for a college quarterback, lacking in all dimensions necessary for the position. I disagree and argue his merits, stressing his leadership and other intangibles. But Phil says it's all bullshit. At one point I threaten to toss him into the swimming pool just beyond the sliding glass door. This sort of talk doesn't impress the girls. They go up to bed, leaving Phil and me to fend for ourselves. Once they're gone, the urge to sleep takes over.

At sunrise I awaken to a splitting headache and a painfully full bladder. Still drunk with the room spinning, I prop myself up and slowly ambulate to the bathroom. I don't know how I manage to get here, but while standing wide-legged in front of the toilet I lose consciousness and my legs turn to jelly. Falling forward, my head strikes a potted plant situated on a shelf above the commode. The contents of the clay pot—dirt and cactus—come crashing down on my head and into the bowl.

After regaining partial consciousness, I finish my business and carry myself, fresh cuts and all, back to the couch where I sleep for three more hours.

Phil and I both awaken to the scream of our kind hostess and the subsequent screaming of her friend. They see my bloody face and assume Phil pummeled me during our spat last night. I laugh at the thought of it, which seems to reassure them.

Relieved, the girls go back upstairs, allowing us some privacy so we can ready ourselves for breakfast. Once the door to the basement closes, it becomes painfully clear that Phil has been cooking up something of his own. He lets out a long squawking fart, smiling as he releases it. It's loud enough for the girls to hear from the floor above. Then there's the stench. It smells inhuman, resembling a mixture of rotten eggs and month-old milk.

Not to be outdone, I counter with an equally violent output.

And so the stage is set for a series of similar volleys. It's like we're having a methane sword fight. If the aroma of flatulence had a visual presence, you wouldn't be able to see your way through the room.

Thankfully, the gasses are pretty well spent by the time Phil and I emerge from the basement, freshly showered and dressed. Our giddy laughter continues through breakfast, but our approaching hangovers on the two hour drive back to Auburn aren't quite so funny.

The concept of doing well academically isn't high on my list of priorities during the first quarter. My course load includes English Composition, Introductory Psychology, World History and Ethics and Society—a class I take along with Phil in order to avoid calculus. This turns out to be an exercise in bad judgment. The two of us use our class time to catch up on social matters and to secretly make fun of the professor, as if we're still in high school.

We agree that he looks like Jackie Gleason without the

hefty girth, and yet he couldn't be more boring. His voice is a singular low tone, and he carries himself around the room like a concrete block. Acting like giddy schoolgirls, Phil and I write notes to each other and sketch caricatures of the professor to keep from falling asleep. Some of the drawings are funny, requiring effort to resist laughing out loud. I picture my mother suffering with boils or some equally bad scenario to keep from busting into hysterics.

But Phil has less self-control. One day he erupts into laughter while the professor is speaking on the ethical perspective of John Stuart Mill, so it's clearly not a case of laughing at the subject matter. The professor wants Phil to explain what could be so funny, asking, "So tell me young man, according to Mill's utilitarianism, how might we approach your antics?"

Phil is dumbstruck. Just like in high school, he has to leave the classroom, which also becomes a funny thing because he's laughing as he's making his way out the door. Again I find myself envying the poor bastard.

It's another case of bad judgment when Phil and I study together for final exams. Most of our efforts take place at the round table in Phil's kitchen with books and notes strewn around the perimeter. A Domino's pizza and a two liter bottle of Diet Coke serve as the table's centerpiece. We start our studying at 9 P.M., and at midnight we ingest Vivarin tablets to assure our alertness. By four o'clock we convince each other that we know enough to do well and that surely the professor won't be so bold as to question us on *this or that*. So we omit *this or that*, thinking we're outsmarting the professor. But even so, it's painfully clear that we've just scratched the surface. We're misguided in our belief that we can compress three months worth of material, after three months worth of procrastination, into seven hours. The realization serves as an unpleasant welcome mat into the world of college academics.

Our mutual dedication to Ethics and Society is duly rewarded at grade time, with me receiving a mark of D+ and Phil registering an F. With the fresh sting of these grades, we pledge never to enroll in the same class again or, if unavoidable, to sit far away from each other.

On a mid-December morning, after the last day of finals, Phil and I drive back in tandem to Fort Lauderdale for the holidays. I finish the quarter with a C average and I'm lucky for it, but it's nothing to be proud of. I promise myself to settle down next term. I'll have to sacrifice some of the partying, and I consider the idea of dropping out of the fraternity.

But before any of that I have to contend with the lawyers. They've held off the deposition until my return, and now they're making me wait until after Christmas. It'll be tough to enjoy the time off with that hanging over my head.

4

B Y far the priciest Christmas gift I receive is the watch my father gave me. It has the name *Tudor* embossed on the orange faceplate, but the brochure says that it's part of the Rolex family of watches. It looks like royalty to me. The only problem is that my damn wrists are too thin. It's the first thing I'd change about my appearance if I could. I want lead pipes for wrists, but instead they look like twin broomsticks wrapped in masking tape. The watch looks clumsy and out of place. I sort of wish I never got it in the first place.

Several days after Christmas Phil and I prepare for the now familiar trek back to Auburn for winter quarter. I'm restless and ready to leave Fort Lauderdale after the fullness of the holiday season. I spent too much time loafing around, letting my brain vegetate. The only day of productive activity was at the deposition where I was picked apart like roadkill in the land of buzzards. None of the attorneys seemed to buy my story. After the interrogation ended, I was sent to an examination room where a legal aide sized my right arm with a tape measure. Arm bent, elbow sticking out, the distance barely surpassed the established length of the side-view mirror combined with the width of the door. It's hard to argue with physical evidence such as this and, realizing the obvious, I stopped trying.

My urge to get away is strong. It's good to know that Auburn is there ready for my return. But even that thought does little to comfort me. I'm haunted by the memory of Lois and her bicycle. I get flashbacks of the scene, which seem like a movie. I can see the orange terry cloth fabric of her shorts and the fairness of her freckled skin, and then I see the 10-speed bicycle lying on the grass a few feet away, front wheel still spinning. Lois lies in the fetal position with her head down against the gray asphalt. Thick red blood dribbles from her head onto her hair and forms a puddle on the road.

Dreams feature me spinning down a spiral, sinking into quicksand or falling from a high perch into the ocean. And even though I'm a decent swimmer in real life I can barely keep my head above water in my dreams.

The most bothersome thing is the insomnia that I've developed. I don't tell anyone about it, figuring it'll go away in time. But a health related matter I can't keep secret is my chronic runny nose. I treat it with the antihistamines my father sent up, but they don't seem to work very well. One afternoon while sitting in the basement of Haley Center, trying to study between wiping my nose, I can't ignore an argument between two students. One calls the other a "snot-nosed punk," and I wonder if he's thinking of me as he says it.

Back at the apartment, Flash and I notice a disturbing smell coming from an unknown place. We both recall a mild odor before the holiday break but were too busy studying for finals to investigate it. Now, with four weeks to intensify during our absence, the smell is overpowering. Mark and Fred are concerned as well and seem equally puzzled as to the source of the stench. Because it permeates the entire apartment there's no way to identify where it's coming from. In a rare moment of teamwork, we agree to clean the entire dwelling together.

Though we're all motivated to dispense with the stink, I'm concerned that Fred and Mark don't share my sense of urgency. While Flash and I clean the bathroom and our bedroom with attention to detail, I notice Fred and Mark slacking off in their efforts to clean the kitchen. Soon they announce they're finished and that the smell is almost gone. But I'm not so convinced. I think all they've done is succeed in masking the odor with an assortment of cleaning products and an air freshener.

A few days pass and, sure enough, the smell is back to full strength. This time we decide to air the apartment out with fans and open windows, despite the fact that we're dealing with temperatures in the upper 30's. After this is accomplished, we enjoy a day or two of relative relief from the foulness.

But once again, sure as the rising sun, the smell returns to haunt us. Now there's a feeling of hopelessness among my suitemates, and it changes our lifestyles because none of us want to invite guests over. The only one who'll stay in the place without complaining is Fred.

One afternoon after class I'm alone in the apartment, washing dishes at the kitchen sink. To scrub away a stubborn region of grime, I open the cabinet door under the sink to get a scouring pad. Instantly, I'm overtaken by an odor so foul my breathing stops. I reflexively shut the cabinet door and run out of the apartment to catch my breath.

Outside on the cold grass, I wonder what the fuck is in there. It's the most abusive olfactory assault I've ever experienced, and I'm pissing mad about it. I let out a string of obscenities in full voice to summon my courage before returning to face the hideous task.

Holding my breath the whole time, I reach down and remove the culprit. It's a badly saturated bag of trash stowed behind the trap pipe of the sink. I can't fathom the rot that must be in there. All I can say is that it's a form of biological weaponry.

I vaguely remember Fred keeping a trash bag near his bed last quarter for the sake of convenience. Rather than taking the filled bag to the dumpster or placing it in the large wastebasket in the kitchen—independent of the cabinet—he must've put it under the sink, back behind the drain with apparently no recall of doing so.

Now Fred denies all connection to the stored trash bag. Meanwhile, he's becoming even more reclusive, and he barely ever talks to me. It gives me a bad feeling, but I don't say anything. I could forgive him, but it's hard when he won't even admit a single degree of blame. I want him to confess and apologize, and I'm holding out for him to do so.

There's a growing intolerance building inside me. Soon it'll go beyond Fred and the annoyance of bad smells.

My classes for winter quarter are World History, English Composition, Introduction to the Physical Sciences and Sociology, which are all standard freshman fare for a liberal arts student. My approach is more disciplined than last quarter. I commit a block of time most evenings for study. After doing a decent amount of coursework, I reward myself by reading articles in *Car and Driver* and *Stereo Review*. Or I watch TV, switching back and forth between *Late Night with David Letterman* and MTV with the irresistible charms of Martha Quinn.

Up to this point, I doubt my college experience differs much from the tens of thousands of other freshmen around the country. But during the third week of January 1984, something changes in the way I see the world. It starts with the course material I'm studying. First, I notice the subject matter becoming more intense and pertinent to the things going on in my life. It's as if some outside force is shaping the material for maximum effect on me personally. And then without effort, I start to form bridges across different fields of study. I merge the physical sciences with sociology and politics, and I look for deeper connections as well. Standard distinctions are washed out by a more unified vision of wholeness. I'm compelled to explore this wholeness.

I take a concept from world history, like the uprising of colonial peoples against a ruling nation, and turn it into a global outcry for personal freedom. This in itself seems harmless. And yet the trouble starts when I begin to see *all* human action throughout history and across cultures as a cry for greater freedom. My thoughts then shift to the notion of dark forces, both within and outside us, cracking down on our freedom. I examine some of the systems imposing their force on us, like the government, the educational system and the corporate world, and decide that their central purpose is to crack down on freedom. Oppression is what all systems are about, and the lowly workers in these systems are either too stupid or too brainwashed to realize what's going on. So they're part of the problem.

Most of the people walking around campus are like robots, behaving and speaking and thinking as if pre-programmed. An ominous force, like Big Brother, is pulling the strings. But unlike Orwell's singular vision of Big Brother, there's a vast array of subtle forces lulling us to sleep. Sleep is the enemy. Vigilance is the only way to fight off the effect.

Reagan is one of these seemingly benign forces working to cement the mass ignorance of the country. His velvety speeches seduce us into being fat and happy and unquestioning. Now I see Flash's allegiance to our president as a sign of his suppression to numb complacency. He's fallen to the dark forces. And this makes him dangerous. It's best to avoid him.

At first I try to keep these thoughts to myself. But it doesn't take long for the stuff to leak out. Most people are turned off by what I have to say. This to me means they've been brainwashed. Within a few days, I think there's no one I can trust, maybe not even Phil.

5

O N Saturday, January 21, I experience what I consider a profound revelation. After being up nearly the entire night, writing and buzzing with energy, I greet the morning feeling ecstatic. I have this vision of harmony among all people of the world in which everyone understands each other intuitively without the need for words. It seems perfectly real, as if the Auburn campus and the rest of planet Earth changed overnight.

Along with this vision of world unity, there's also a stunning array of sounds, colors and comforting feelings passing through me as I lie in bed. The images come and go like clouds overhead, but faster than clouds and harder to keep up with. I know they can't be the products of my feeble brain. They must come from another place. My mind is like a radio, pulling in a vast stream of signals, and I have the ability to tune the stream into something sensible.

Because of their clarity and joyful nature I think the messages must be coming from God, as if He is broadcasting to my radio brain. I'm grateful to be the receiver, and I wonder how many other people are privy to such wisdom. How could I distinguish these people from the rest? I want to know the answer, but above all I want to remain in this state of happy clarity. This must be what heaven is like.

No one else in the apartment is up yet, but when they are they'll greet a new reality. And I'm convinced that they'll be better for it.

By mid-morning I'm out of bed, eager to explore my surroundings. Walking around the apartment, I find that even the most mundane things around me have gained special significance and symbolic value. Simple things translate into a message of wholeness, like the shape of a faucet or the way plates are arranged on the table.

Songs hold the strongest symbolic pull, and I find myself craving music as if it's a pipeline to the Great Messenger. After getting dressed I sit and watch MTV in a spellbound state. Michael Jackson, U2 and The Police draw me into their spell. I notice that the Moon is a prominent feature on TV this morning, and it becomes a focal point for me. The Moon is more than just a satellite orbiting Earth. It's a living being transmitting important messages.

Not wanting my family to miss out on this wisdom, I decide to call them right away. First, I call my dad who's home watching something else on television. Instead of getting into the normal preliminary phone chat, I tell him right off that he needs switch the channel to MTV, which I know he's never watched before. I tell him to pay special attention to the Moon when it shows up on the screen.

Then I call my mother's house, hoping to give her the same advice, but instead I get my sister Julia on the other end. "Watch MTV," I tell her with urgency, "you're gonna get messages from the Moon." Both she and my father do as they're told, but they don't seem to get the same thrilling results.

Once the euphoria passes through me, a new disturbance

comes to the fore. It starts when Flash comes home after shopping for food. He asks why I'm so preoccupied with the television, which isn't typical for me. Then he mentions how I've been acting strange over the past few days, and he asks if there's anything wrong.

"No, there's nothing wrong," I say. Then I tell him about the newfound wisdom I've received, compliments of the Moon. This prompts a smirk from Flash, which adds to my defensiveness. After he leaves the room, I lock the door and prop a chair against the doorknob so no one can enter. Then, for an additional measure of safety, I move one of the large metal desks to block the window.

Alone in the bedroom with the television blaring MTV, I take out a pocketknife and carve the words THE MOON RULES on the lacquered door.

Soon Flash and a few others approach the door and demand I open it. I won't budge and say so with confidence. But it scares me to think of them plowing through or busting through the window. "Get the hell away!" I yell from behind the barricade.

They ignore me and remain close to the door, discussing how to extract me. I accuse them of being agents of the devil. I think they want to torture or kill me for my newfound knowledge. Knowing it'll only be a matter of minutes before they harness the strength to get in, I decide to leave at once.

I put on a jacket to fend off the cold, then pull back the desk from the lone bedroom window. Since no one has come around yet to the back of the apartment, I can dash for the parking lot undetected. I get into my El Camino and screech the tires.

It's an overcast day with intermittent sprinkles and a mild breeze. It can't be much above freezing. I drive around the outskirts of town on unfamiliar roads while checking the rearview mirror almost as much as the view ahead. Flash or the cops must be trying to hunt me down.

Looking for a deserted location I happen upon the Auburn Industrial Park, which has no sign of life on a Saturday. After searching the area I drive into the lot of the Rus Uniform Company and select a spot next to a big delivery van, keeping me hidden from the access road.

For the better part of the day, I sit in my car listening to the stereo blast out tunes. At intervals, I crank the engine to heat up the cabin and to keep the battery from going dead, which may be my only concession to the practicalities of life. Otherwise, I'm consumed by the messages being offered up by the radio. It's as if the disc jockey is talking to me personally. Either what he's saying targets my thinking, or maybe my brain is molding around his statements. I can't tell which.

Later, it's the voice of a female disc jockey, sounding like she's sexed-up just for me. She says something suggestive, then plays a song that confirms her desire for me. The song says what we'll do together and where we'll do it.

The euphoria from the morning is back again. But depending on the programming of the radio station I'm listening to, my mood shifts with each song. At least twice over the course of the afternoon I hear *Sunday Bloody Sunday* by U2. I think it means there'll be a revolution or a worldwide transformation taking place on Sunday, tomorrow. This is big news. Then there are other songs that seem to be describing me right now as I am, sitting here in the car. One is *Owner of a Lonely Heart* by Yes and the other is *King of Pain* by The Police.

The notion of time plays a big part in my thinking. I get the idea that in the near future, maybe tomorrow—Bloody Sunday, after all—we'll enter a universe where time has no meaning. Past, present and future will compress together into a wavy strand of infinity. I don't understand the mechanics involved or what purpose it's supposed to serve, but I take it as prophecy nonetheless.

This idea of timelessness turns into an overpowering belief as the afternoon progresses, leading me to toss my new Tudor watch out the window, beyond the parking lot and into the woods. Since the watch came from my father, I think of my gesture as a victory over the limiting world of Father Time. By tossing the watch into the woods I'm putting Father Time into Mother Earth, which is where I think he belongs. Now I can enter timelessness without corruption.

As darkness spreads over the plains of East Alabama I venture back to the CDV apartment complex, feeling rejuvenated and far less paranoid than when I left. It's Saturday night, time to celebrate the coming transformation.

Back at the apartment I explain to Flash that everything is fine. I don't argue over the strangeness of my behavior or the so-called "crap" I scratched into the door. When he asks where I've been all day, I tell him I've been on an important mission and leave it at that.

Tonight there's a big party at the fraternity house. To prepare I take a long shower, and it's a euphoric sensation having the warm water massage my skin. When I turn off the faucet I hear knocking and complaining from the other side of the bathroom door, saying I've been in here for nearly an hour. I think of how ignorant these people are with their intrusiveness and petty ways.

Once dressed I join Phil and a few others to go to the frat house. I feel as though something big will happen there tonight—the end of one world era and the beginning of a new way. I'm happy to be at the forefront of this transition. But beneath the happy feeling there's a gnawing agitation starting to emerge. I wonder if something isn't quite right after all.

I want to go to the party right now, but we're delayed by one of the guys who's on the phone, taking his sweet time.

To show my disapproval I do a roundhouse kick, smashing through the kitchen window.

"That's not cool," says the guy on the phone.

"What the hell'dya do that for?" Phil asks.

I tell him that windows won't be necessary in the near future without explaining further. It doesn't go over well with Phil, but he keeps quiet about it. He probably thinks I'm drunk or stoned or both.

We show up at the ATO house for what's known as their annual Beach Party. As if to scoff at the cold weather, the brothers have chosen the third weekend in January to pay tribute to the sunny days of summer. The thermostat in the house is turned up to simulate the desired seasonal change, and beach balls are strewn along the hallways. A group of brothers dumped a truckload of sand onto the floor of the dining hall where they set up a volleyball net and a lifeguard chair. Some of the partygoers are dressed in bathing attire and Hawaiian lei's, but they're in the minority. There's a rum punch concoction going around and music blaring throughout the house—mostly summertime tunes. And like all ATO parties there's a keg of cold beer in the lobby.

Most of the brothers and pledges are here, along with the little sisters and a good number of non-Greek students. It's one of the better attended parties of the year, despite the fact that there's no live band playing.

Early on I join in kicking beach balls up and down the hallway, taking care not to hit anyone carrying a beer. A short while later, I'm in the dining hall dancing in the sandpit. When the song *Burning Down the House* comes on, I take it as an invitation to set the fraternity house ablaze. Borrowing a lighter from one of the smokers, I set flame to a wooden chair and hope for a dramatic effect.

It's not the kind of chair that goes up easily. After a few frustrating trials I let go of the idea. But my need to destroy something is strong. So I pitch the chair backward over my shoulder and kick a hole in the door to the chapter room.

Now I've got everyone's attention.

One of the older brothers, with the illustrious name Sterling, escorts me to an overstuffed chair in the formal chapter room to talk about what's going on. It's quieter now, and there's a cluster of brothers standing around us in case I get another violent urge.

Sterling talks to me in a gentle way, which has a calming effect. He's like a wise prophet who's progressed beyond the need for violence or dramatic displays. His words of assurance lead me to think he knows what I'm going through, like he's traveled the same road. I thank him for the advice, figuring I may need to talk with him again.

Meanwhile the house starts emptying out. It's amazing how quickly a little fire and vandalism can suck the life out of a party. Much calmer now, I decide to go along with Phil, Deano and a few of the brothers to the Hungry Hunter nightclub, which is on the highway connecting Auburn to the slightly larger town of Opelika. As the name suggests, the club is a pickup joint. With roughly equal parts students and locals, it's a popular place to be on a Saturday night.

Sitting in the passenger seat of Phil's Celica, I look up at the nearly full Moon then down at the series of headlights from oncoming traffic. Looking back and forth between the Moon and the headlights, I sense a connection between these sources of light. Suddenly it hits me that the Moon is God, or at the very least the eye of God, and the headlights on the highway are transmitting His messages for everyone. What a thrilling discovery! It takes a supreme act of self-control not to blurt it out in the car.

We arrive at the crowded bar and order longneck Budweisers all around. Without a table available we stand in a circle, looking for people we might know. Occasionally, a pair of us takes a walk around the club, scanning for attractive girls. During one such round with Deano, I start telling him about my new insights. But he can't hear what I'm saying over the blaring dance songs and the loud chatter of people. It's a repetition of me yelling and Deano saying "what?"

I signal for us to go outside where we can hear each other and where we'll have the added bonus of being in the presence of the Moon. On our way out I borrow Phil's car keys so we can sit in comfort.

I consider Deano an open-minded person who can grasp the deeper meaning of things, despite his tendency to play the fool. So now, with my alert on high, I choose Deano to be the recipient of my compelling revelations. They're so powerful that I have to share them with someone and he's the best choice for now.

My approach takes the form of a religious sermon, fire and brimstone variety, preaching to the unconverted. Sitting in the driver's seat of Phil's car, with the engine running to generate some heat, I tell Deano the truth of the world as I know it. I talk about the mass brainwashing of humanity and how our ignorance will be our undoing. I say there's an urgent need for action if we hope to liberate ourselves. I struggle to explain the great possibilities in front of us and how we'll be helped along, every step of the way, by the Moon. Even when the path seems at its bleakest, the Moon will be here to comfort and guide us, but only if we're open to it.

To demonstrate the Moon's power I turn on the radio, explaining that the next song will impart a message of profound wisdom. The station plays *One Thing Leads to Another* by The Fixx, and I crank it up for better effect. We listen to a few more songs during which I notice Deano getting restless. When I tell him that Michael Jackson's song *Thriller* keeps changing every time I listen to it, he says he's heard enough.

As an act of diplomacy, Deano mentions some common

points between his philosophy and mine. I stay quiet for the moment, until he unleashes a sarcastic attack on the notion of lunar theology by saying, "It's nothin' but a dead rock."

The last thing a preacher wants is for someone to belittle his sermon, so I argue back at Deano, getting more worked up the more I talk. Deano stays calm throughout, telling me to lighten up. But I can't shake my anger. Suddenly we're out of the car arguing in the parking lot.

There's a couple in a nearby car steaming up the windows. They notice Deano and me yelling, so the male counterpart of the couple, a stocky built Native American, cracks open his window to ask what's the matter.

"The Moon is God," I say, "and this asshole won't believe me," pointing to Deano. By now any effort toward tactfulness is beyond me. The Indian looks over at his girlfriend, who starts to laugh, but he doesn't laugh along with her. He tells me that my philosophy is just as plausible as any other, and he goes on to point out how the world's major religions share a lot of the same ideas on the nature of God.

Deano shows a liking for the stranger's way of reasoning. This means I have to make my case to both parties while they gang up on me with standard nonsense I don't want to hear. I'm ready to fire away at both of them.

Without warning I lift my right leg and kick the partially-opened window of the Indian's car, spreading glass across him and his girlfriend. Deano grabs me, but I shake him off. Then when he tries to hold me in place I pin a hard right to his chest, and I kick him as he falls to the ground.

It's time to head back into the club.

I have a murky sense that I've gone over the edge this time. I only hope I can last the night without further incident. But within a few minutes three policemen arrive and they want to know about the broken car window.

One cop gets the story from the Indian and his girlfriend,

while the others stand at the club's entrance to keep me from running away. It doesn't take a degree in psychiatry for the cops to realize that a ride to the Student Health Center is the best plan for me. The bill for the broken window will be sent to my father in Fort Lauderdale.

I arrive at the Drake Student Health Center courtesy of the University Police at around 2 A.M., complaining of hunger. After a quick interview with the nurse on duty, I'm led to a small white room where I wait for food. The only form of sustenance they can offer me at this hour is a bowl of split pea soup, which I accept gratefully.

The nurse brings me a steamy bowl on a hospital tray with crackers. I thank her and sit at the foot of the bed while eating the soup in a state of wonder. It's strange, but my sense of taste is sharper than before, as if all my sensory energy is tuned into the split pea soup and the rest of the world is tuned out. It's the best soup I've ever had, with a perfect blend of flavor and texture. Noticing my delight, the nurse is kind enough to indulge me with a second bowl.

During this second helping, a graduate student counselor named Dante enters the room and asks if he can interview me. He's a courteous, soft-spoken guy with brown curly hair matted to one side from sleeping. It's a bad case of bedhead. He explains he was wakened for the purpose of seeing me and that it might take him a few minutes to regain his alertness. I jokingly ask him about the *Inferno*, given his namesake, and whether he came from there. He laughs at this. Then, not joking, I ask him if God made the split pea soup, which makes him laugh again. He lets both questions go unanswered.

Having decided he means no harm, I tell Dante about the powerful images and ideas I've been having. He tries to take notes, but it's hard for him to keep up. I figure the notes will go directly to God once Dante polishes them up, so I slow

down to let him to record them better. After a while he stops
writing altogether and lets me talk about whatever I want. This
makes me think the test is over—the test of God's judgment,
that is—and I've passed. I've gained admission into a special
group. Something makes me think that it's an elite celestial
group, like a gallery of prophets.

An image appears in my mind of an entourage of prophets
guiding me along the path to oneness. Our first meeting will
be held in Atlanta at an all-night diner where we'll talk over
coffee and a wide assortment of breakfast dishes. I picture the
diner decorated in gaudy orange with wall-to-wall carpeting,
and there we are sitting at a large round table. After consuming
the food we'll take up the agenda of the pre-dawn hour, which
is how to enlighten people with the assistance of the Moon.
Nothing could be more important than this.

It's a vivid image playing joyfully in my brain. In the scene,
Dante is sitting next to me at the table. He's my guide. He'll
help smooth over the unfamiliar protocol.

"When do we leave for Atlanta?" I ask.

He tells me to get some rest first, and then he wishes me
good night. He says he'll be back in the morning, first thing.
Before leaving, he hands me a hospital gown that looks like it
might fit someone half my size.

I'll be alone for the rest of the night, but I don't feel alone.
Instead, I think God is watching over me with renewed interest. It's a comforting feeling, and I want to look good in His
eyes, so I take extra pains to be on my best behavior. I fold my
clothes in an exacting way, and I negotiate the awkward hospital gown with the closest I can come to serenity.

In the small connecting bathroom I discover a miniature
tube of toothpaste with a generic toothbrush alongside it.
There's a fresh towel, a washcloth and a stack of miniature
Dixie cups. The place is immaculate. It's as if this room has
always been here for me, awaiting my occupancy whenever I

was ready. Now the time has come.

After the bathroom ritual, I turn off the light, tuck myself into the small bed and say a little prayer to God, as if we're longtime buddies. It's my first prayer in years.

My sleep is packed with a flood of images, some of them beautiful, some funny, which at one point causes me to wake up in a fit of laughter. A nurse knocks on the door to see if everything is okay.

"Yes, I'm fine," I say, wondering if I should invite her in. Maybe we could have a little party in here. But it's probably better to get a good night's sleep. My energy will be needed for the next step of the journey.

6

As the sun rises to dimly light the room, a nurse
knocks on the door and tells me I should shower and
get ready for a trip to the hospital. She says I'll be
transported to the East Alabama Medical Center, which is the
closest hospital in neighboring Opelika. I get up and do as she
says, thinking this must be a part of the grand plan.

Dante arrives with a simple tray for breakfast—juice, a roll
and a small bowl of oatmeal—not quite the banquet I envi-
sioned last night. While I'm eating, Dante tells me that the
hospital is the most appropriate place for me to go. There I can
get proper round-the-clock attention. He says everything will
be fine and that he doesn't expect me to be there very long.

Somewhere in his speech, I read between the lines that I'm
going to the hospital to have sex with a select woman. It must
be a prelude to the gallery of prophets. This thought pleases
me and it assures my cooperation with his plan. Dante says
nothing to discourage my new belief. Maybe he senses it's the
only way I'll go without a fight.

Like last night, I sit in the backseat of a University Police car with two officers up front. Dante follows behind in his car. The campus is quiet on a Sunday morning, with just one lone jogger on Magnolia Avenue dressed in sweats. It's cold out, and I can see the jogger's breath. We approach the center of town turning left at Toomer's Drugstore.

Traveling out of town on the Auburn-Opelika Highway, we pass the Hungry Hunter on the right side of the road. My thoughts drift to Deano and the Indian, and I wonder if they're aware of how ignorant they were last night. I'm lost in thoughts of this sort until we approach the emergency entrance to the hospital.

Flanked by the two cops and Dante leading the way, I'm ushered to a small examining room. The first nurse to see me is an attractive yet husky brown haired woman in her early 40's. She's not exactly what I had in mind, but I figure she's the woman I'll be having sex with.

She asks me a lot of irrelevant questions, such as, "Are you currently taking any medications?" "Have you had any operations or serious injuries?" and so on. Then she reads off a bunch of illnesses, to which I'm supposed to answer "yes" or "no." She asks about my legal history and past drug use and says she wants to get an idea of my family upbringing.

I give her all the information in a perfunctory way, but rattle off my own stream of thoughts when given the chance. The nurse looks restless when I shift to the topic of sex, which seems strange to me. Doesn't she know the plan?

Not wanting to waste anymore time, I tell her that sex is not nearly as dirty as she might think. Then I invite her to have sex with me—once Dante leaves the room, that is. She declines, but thanks me anyway. Maybe she would've agreed if Dante weren't here.

After writing a note in my newly created chart, Dante says he has to go. This is unexpected, and I'm sad to see him leave. I thought he would guide me through my whole stay and wait outside during the sex. Before saying goodbye, he assures me he'll be back for visits.

My next destination is another examination room in the adult psychiatric ward of the hospital, which is on the ground floor. Here they take a series of measurements—blood pressure, respiration, height, weight and the drawing of blood and urine to glean more data. A blonde nurse with acne tells me to strip down so she can check for bruises and other such things. I wonder why all the fuss, but then a new thought comes to mind. I realize that these tests are essential in order to match me with the appropriate woman. I figure my soul mate hasn't been located yet, but soon she'll be brought to me with the aid of these tests. Maybe the friendly policemen who brought me here will track her down and bring her to me. Suddenly, everything makes sense. My cooperation will be necessary.

After the admitting procedures are complete, I'm escorted to a formal office. It's the first one I've seen with carpeting. There's an impressive oak desk and an array of framed diplomas and certificates displayed on the wall across the door. This is the office of Dr. Jenkins, chief psychiatrist, who's been assigned to oversee my treatment.

With the sudden change in scenery and its new air of formality, I forget about the sexual plans in store for me. I wonder how this meeting is supposed to fit the plan. It's the first awareness that I'm not in charge, and it makes me restless.

Dr. Jenkins introduces himself while his eyes are focused downward on my chart. With his hands busy writing, a handshake between us isn't an option. He asks questions to discern whether I'm aware of my surroundings and if I know the current date. He asks me who the president is and has me memorize some unrelated words.

The entire interview takes about five minutes, resulting in a note in my chart stating that I'm a *19-year-old, white, male AU student with progressive agitation, confusion and loss of control.* Then Dr. Jenkins writes a prescription for the drug Loxitane, 25 milligrams, to be taken orally four times per day. Further instructions state that if I refuse to take it orally, I am to get it in the form of an intramuscular injection.

Immediately thereafter, at the nurse's station, I get my first dose.

The head nurse and an orderly give me a tour of the unit, stopping at the private room where I'll be staying. It's two doors down from the nurse's station, next to a place they call the seclusion room. On the other side of the hall is the men's shower and bathroom. To get to the large meeting room—or day room, as they call it—you have to go back past the nurse's station and then past the main entrance. The day room functions as the place for meals, activities and group therapy. Right now the place reeks of cigarette smoke. Just before entering the day room you find the office of Dr. Jenkins and, across from him, the office of my assigned counselor, a man named Terry.

After the tour the nurse hands me a written summary of the rules of the unit along with a schedule of meals and daily activities. Knowing I won't read the stuff, she also gives an oral presentation of everything there on the paper. I'm told to read over the material again if I get confused. When the nurse asks if I have any questions, my mind is blank. Pleased by the progress we're making so far, she smiles and rises to leave. Now I can settle into my new surroundings, keeping mindful of the rules.

A young attendant is assigned to keep an eye on me and chart my actions every 30 minutes. He's a short, pudgy, Hispanic looking guy in his mid-20's who never says anything except to tell me when I'm doing something wrong.

On this first morning I wander around the unit, going from one patient's room to another. The pudgy guy says I'm not supposed to go into other patients' rooms unless invited, but I ignore him and keep wandering, investigating the place for eligible women. Soon the head nurse comes over and gives me a tougher warning. I obey for a while, but once she's out of my visual field I go back to my wandering ways.

A new feeling of sluggishness hits me, and I have to lie down. Deciding that any bed will do for now, I lie down on the nearest freshly made bed, which apparently isn't the one assigned to me. The pudgy guy tells me I have to get up, to which I say in return, "Get the hell out of here."

This he does, but soon comes back armed with the head nurse at his side. She gives me the same order and marches me down the hall to the seclusion room, which I figure is just a normal private room. As I sit on the bed I can hear the door being locked from the other side.

The seclusion room is a small, L-shaped box with nothing in it but a hospital bed. It has a massive wooden door with a tiny peephole at eye level. I try looking out through the hole, but can't see anything because it's designed for others to look in. I also bang at the door with all the force I can muster, but it's not budging. For greater impact, I back up and charge at the door, leading first with one shoulder and then the other. It's a futile exercise—a self-defeating sequence of running, smashing and writhing in pain. The solid door remains intact. Yelling at the staff doesn't do much good either.

Soon I'm worn out from the medication and the expenditure of energy. After an hour or so in the room, I'm overcome by exhaustion. I lie down to get some rest and find that the goddamn bed is too short. I commence wrestling with the sheet in search of a comfortable position, fearing all the while that I'll fall off either side onto the cold linoleum floor. After a few minutes of relative stillness, I feel cold and start to shiver. This room could serve as a meat locker when they aren't using it to store live human bodies. I search around for a blanket, but there's nothing except for the bleached white sheets, thin as paper.

Now I feel tormented from all sides and my frustration grows to rage. I start hurling out insults, begging for someone to bring me a fucking blanket. The yelling itself is energizing, calling forth a barrage of cottonmouthed, foam-spewing profanity—the more vile the better. I picture the people on the other side of the door shrinking and melting from the wickedness of my words.

Soon the door opens, which prompts me to stop yelling. A young black nurse tosses me a blanket from the entryway. Here's an olive branch I can accept. I feel calmer now, but also ashamed, like a spoiled brat on a tirade. After the shame subsides, I think of how remarkable it was that this beautiful nurse risked her life to bring me a blanket. God bless her. With that thought, I drift into a fitful sleep.

At around noon I hear the sound of the door opening again, awakening me to the unmistakable smell of fried chicken. It's on a food tray being delivered by the same lovely nurse, my savior, who's wearing a cream colored outfit instead of the standard white or blue. With a pleasant smile, she rolls the tray table to my bed and says to enjoy the food. But first she has medication to give me, which I willingly take as a tribute to her kindness. She smiles again and leaves the room, locking the door behind her.

By this time I'm famished, and it seems I've got a craving for everything on the tray. How could they know that this is exactly what I wanted? I plunge into the meal, eating everything remotely edible. There's fried chicken, green beans, mashed potatoes with gravy, some kind of warm apple dessert and hot tea, which is room temperature by the time I get to it. The meal is gratifying beyond measure, even more than the split pea soup last night. It now seems that everything I've endured up to this point has been a necessary trial, designed by

God, which will soon be over. This meal is a testament to the fact that God is here, watching over me with loving eyes.

The only things I leave on the tray are the chicken bones and the packets of salt and pepper. Somehow these condiments have deeper significance to me than usual. To further explore their meaning, I clear an area on the synthetic wood surface of the tray table and pour the contents into separate piles. It occurs to me that the two piles of seasoning represent the Light and the Dark, the Caucasian and the African, the Alpha and the Omega. I begin to think that here is the place where the polar forces of the world can be reconciled.

It's an invigorating thought, surely part of God's test. I now realize what I must do. I have to merge the two piles into one. This is why I'm here—to save humanity from annihilation. Destroy the boundary between and unite. Time is crucial. I have to do this right away, before we exterminate ourselves.

I mix the contents together and dab my finger into the pile for a taste. As I'm doing this, there's a knock on the door followed by the presence of an unfamiliar person who comes in and rolls away the tray table. My universe, embodied in grains of salt and pepper, disappears.

By evening I drift in and out of consciousness, groggy from the Loxitane. Somewhere at the bridge between sleep and wakefulness, I conjure up an exciting vision. The scene is in Africa, where I'm on a safari with this stunningly attractive black woman. She's slender, tall and full-breasted, wearing nothing but a semitransparent gown. Her matted hair is long, traveling down to the small of her back near her heavenly hips. She has golden brown eyes and her lips sparkle with moisture.

At first she smiles without saying anything. Then she whispers my name and says she'll come for me soon. She repeats this message two or three times, sounding sweeter with each repetition. It's what I want to hear, possibly the best message I could hear. I ask her what her name is, and she says it's Nikita, or maybe something else starting with the letter N. Whatever it is, I say it over and over again, long after the vision leaves my mind. I wonder how soon it'll be when she arrives, and I pray for her to come now to take me out of this place.

In the midst of these thoughts, I undress and lie naked on top of the bed, thinking this might conjure her back, hopefully in the flesh this time. But it only makes me cold. I put my clothes back on and bundle under the blanket for more sleep.

Late in the evening, a knock and a voice beckon me to the door, jarring me out of a deep slumber. I pull myself up and walk toward the door, using a wall for balance. Arriving at the peephole, I look out to see nothing but a fish-eyed blur. Of course I've looked through the damn hole 50 times prior to this, and each time it's been the same nullifying result.

The nasal voice of a woman asks if I might be ready to leave the seclusion room. Maybe she thinks she's doing me a huge favor by rescuing me from the pit of despair or something. But by now I really don't give a shit. Maybe that's the point—they wait until you don't care about your freedom before they let you out.

I agree to the offer and after some fumbling with keys the door is opened. Across the threshold are three male attendants and the nasal nurse, all eyeing me with apprehension. They're probably thinking I'll attack, and if that's the case they're ready. Though she's trying to conceal it, I can see the nurse hiding a syringe, and one of the guys has a coiled leather strap for God-knows-what-purpose. With Nikita still in mind, my thoughts are far from violent. But the syringe is a threatening sight. I back up toward the bed, telling the nurse I won't take the shot.

The nurse offers a deal, telling me that if I go to my pre-assigned room calmly I could forgo the injection. It's an easy choice. I accept the arrangement while watching my ass the whole time. Nikita is miles away.

7

NEXT morning I awaken to the presence of a breakfast tray and a liquid dose of Loxitane. The nurse watches me hawk-like as I drink the nasty fluid, chasing it down with orange juice. In disgust, I ask the nurse what the drug is supposed to do.

"It's to help you clear your thoughts," she says.

This is too vague an answer for me. I want to know more, but the nurse isn't prepared for this kind of conversation. Her chief concern is that I stick to the Monday morning program—medication, breakfast, then a shower—no deviations permitted.

After the required shower, I walk down the hall with a terrifically stiff neck. It's like nothing I've ever experienced and the pain is unbearable. My head droops back to the right, and it's stuck in this deranged position. I stop midway down the hall, grunting for someone to help.

The charge nurse and a few other people hoist me back to bed while the nurse asks me about the problem. I can barely speak because my mouth has gone bone dry. Here's another situation to contend with. When I do manage to speak, my words are packed with a helpless gloom. It's hard keeping it all inside. Lying down in my paralytic, groggy, dry-mouthed state I start crying like a baby. A second nurse comes in with a shot of Benadryl, which she delivers into my right arm. This has the effect of thrusting me back into sleep.

When I wake up a few hours later, the neck stiffness is gone, thank God, but the cottonmouth is still there and my vision is now blurred. Testing my sight, I can barely make out the image of Dr. Jenkins approaching for a bedside visit.

Getting right to the heart of the matter, he says I had a *dystonic reaction* to the medication, which somehow explains my neck stiffness. And now I'm having *anticholinergic effects*, which account for my current dry mouth and vision problems. He says these are side effects from the Loxitane and, to combat them, he'll need to use a second medication called Cogentin. Dr. Jenkins sounds like the embodiment of confidence as he explains these things. Meanwhile, I feel like a retarded kid.

"Thanks for the information doc," is all I can say.

It's about this time that I meet my assigned therapist, Terry, but I don't remember our first meeting other than fragments of the two of us sitting together in his office. The thing I do most when I'm with him is argue about being hospitalized against my will and how urgent it is that I get out of here. I tell him I'm missing classes and other important engagements. Once this topic is exhausted, I rant about the Moon and God and the anticipated sexual liaison, which somehow got overlooked. In my calmer moments, I tell Terry about my family life and mention the fact that I knocked a woman off her bicycle about six months ago.

But during the first few days, it's mostly a matter of him convincing me I need to stay in the hospital. At one point he says, "You're not well," which may be accurate but still tough to swallow. Mostly I don't accept it. My version is more like, *It's you and the goddamn world that aren't well, and now I can see the light.* But this thought and the ability to say it aren't in alignment. I can barely find my ass with two hands.

In the back of my mind I suspect Terry might be right about me, but to admit it would be devastating. It would mean that all the compelling and beautiful images I've been seeing, and my idea of world unity, are nothing but meaningless mirages constructed by a sick mind. To accept Terry's version of reality, I'd have to turn my back on the most enlightening thoughts I've ever had. And I'd have to admit that I'm the sick one. This is not something I can easily do, not with the evidence as I see it.

When we aren't arguing about my mental state or where I need to be, I can see the good in Terry. His voice is gentle without judgement, and he's interested in hearing what I have to say. There's a kind of serenity about him, even during the moments when I'm ready to combust into flames of rage. In fact, he's always calm. Putting out fires is his gift.

Terry has a couple of nicknames for me, each one complimentary. The one he uses most is Big Guy. He says it like we're old pals or teammates on the football field. "Hey Big Guy." I like hearing him say it.

My daily routine includes a 50 minute meeting with Terry, followed by a brief meeting with Dr. Jenkins, who isn't much for doling out the compassion, at least not in my case. He has this air of detached confidence, like a man on a mission. His goal is to remove the patient's sickness, and he has one method of doing it. Talking with the patient is hardly necessary for the job, so I see him for no more than five to ten minutes, which is all he needs to check my symptoms. He could probably get all the necessary information from the chart or the head nurse, but that might call into question his professional ethics. What matters to him is the Loxitane, which he started at 100 milligrams on the first day and, despite the obnoxious side effects, he increases to 200 milligrams by day three. His methods don't include informing the patient ahead of time about side effects, and it doesn't really matter whether the patient is willing to take the drug. You must take it—either orally or in the ass—it's as simple as that. The doctor knows best.

I've met a fellow patient named Neil. He's a docile looking man of about 30 who wears horn-rimmed glasses with thick lenses bulging out beyond the frames. His voice is soft and timid, but what he lacks in vocal presence he makes up for in endurance. Neil can talk for hours on matters big and small, not caring whether he repeats himself. For some reason he chooses me to be the primary recipient of his verbal fodder, maybe because he has exhausted the will of the other patients and staff. But it doesn't bother me. I could use some attention.

We have meals together in the day room, where we tackle the gamut of issues as we see them. Here's my chance to share the insights popping into my head without being ignored or coddled or told that I'm sick. It's like an inoculation against the strong arm of the staff and the drugs. With Neil I can keep alive my idea of bringing oneness to the world, even while everyone else considers it delusional folly.

Late one morning I gather up my things to take a shower. I haven't seen Neil yet today and I'm bored, figuring a shower might refresh me. I've been wearing the same old clothes since my arrival four days ago—faded blue jeans and a brown polo shirt. They're not dirty because the staff launders them during the night shift while I sleep in a gown.

Walking down the hall with my towel, clothes and toiletries in hand, I approach the men's bathroom. I open the door and put my things on a chair, but then realize I'm not the only one in here. Without thinking, I look over at the bathtub in the corner, and there in plain view is Neil with his eyes shut, stroking his erect penis. "Holy shit!" I say as I dart red-faced out of the bathroom, leaving my personal items behind.

Later in the day, the head nurse tells me I have to move from my private room into a dorm style room with four beds. She says there's a new patient arriving who needs a private room. So in a matter of a few minutes my meager belongings are transferred to the bed situated diagonally across from Neil's. I'm not happy about losing the private room, but it's good to have a friendly face nearby. And it's good that Neil's bed isn't directly next to mine in case he gets the urge to jerk himself off under the sheets.

On Sunday, January 29th, the Los Angeles Raiders crush the Washington Redskins in Superbowl XVIII, but I don't even bother to watch the game. Normally I wouldn't miss a Superbowl, but these aren't normal times. I spend the day in bed.

With only a handful of staff on the unit during weekends, no one comes in to push activities on us. Neil and I and another male patient occupy our beds in the dorm for the better part of the day. We talk for a while and then lie silent. But then a curious thing happens that I can't explain away. In the midst of lying there in silence, a wave of laughter hits all three of us at the same time. Then the laughter dies down and we're silent again for a while.

But soon it happens again, all three of us at once bursting into hysterics. It's synchronized, spontaneous laughter and it's amazingly fun. When it's done we don't say anything about it, as if it's an everyday sort of thing.

Looking back on it, you could say that one of us started laughing and then the other two, being suggestible and in good spirits already, caught the wave and went with it. But that doesn't seem like what happened. It felt like the three of us were tuning in to the same subliminal broadcast, funny to us all. I don't know which is the right explanation. All I know is that it's the first and the last time this ever happened to me and it was exhilarating. I doubt the Superbowl was as entertaining.

The very next day Neil tells me he's leaving the hospital to return to his hometown, which is some place in New Jersey. Realizing Neil has difficulty separating fact from fiction, I don't really believe him. He's like a fixture in the psychiatric ward if ever there was one, and it's unthinkable to me that he should be anywhere but here. He's reliable company, a part of the daily routine. I can't imagine him leaving.

But his mother shows up later in the day to retrieve him. Neil carries a small suitcase, his mother walking alongside, when he approaches me in the day room to say goodbye. At last it dawns on me—he's really leaving. We exchange phone numbers and I invite him to visit me in Fort Lauderdale sometime, maybe over spring break. His mother tells me they'll think about it, but I can tell she's only humoring me. She and Neil wish me well.

I can't look at them when I say goodbye.

8

IN addition to counseling me individually, Terry phones my parents in Florida to give them regular updates on my status. My mother is frantic about the whole ordeal and requires a lot of emotional support, while my father stays calm, preferring to stick with the practical aspects of my care. Apparently my mother was planning to jump on a plane and see me on the first day of my admission. But she was advised to wait until I'm more stabilized.

Personally I don't see any reason for my parents to come up here on account of my being hospitalized. I figure I'll be getting out of this hellhole soon. It's a big misunderstanding as far as I can tell. On the phone I tell both of them that I'm not really sick, despite what the staff says, and that soon I can resume classes with only a few days to catch up on coursework. I add that my being in the hospital is some kind of test, designed by God.

This test can be tiring though, and I hope it'll be over soon. When it's finally done, the least they can do is throw me a party after all the shit I've gone through. Figuring God to be a trickster, He'll probably make it a surprise party, throwing it when I least expect it. So I keep guessing—*when will it be?* When someone asks me to come to the day room, or when I go to see Terry in his office, I find myself thinking *maybe this is it.* A representative of God and the staff and my friends will pop into view and yell, "Surprise!" Then we'll all have a good laugh. Once the party's over I'll go back to my classes at Auburn, and the professors will understand my absence. Heck, they might even be in on it. Maybe I'll get some sort of plaque or certificate of achievement for my successful efforts. I'll hang it over my bed at CDV, next to the calendar with the sports cars.

But Jesus this is getting to be one hell of an elaborate test. Think of it—a mock psychiatric ward complete with nurses, aides, a psychiatrist and drugs with side effects. What's the point of all this orchestration? There has to be something deeper, something of significance going on here. I try to figure it out, and for a short time the ideas align themselves to make it all seem reasonable. But my powers of creativity are slipping away.

Somewhere in the midst of this mindset, my mother arrives. I'm sitting alone on my bed barefoot, unshaven and wearing the familiar attire when I see my mother coming forward to greet me. Standing behind her is a friend of hers from church named Pat who also has a son attending Auburn. Fortunately for Pat, her son has all his marbles intact.

Noticing my mother approaching, I wonder why she's here, and I then see Pat standing behind her. What could this mean? Ignoring their greetings, I demand that they take me back to CDV, telling them I need to get back to class and be done with this bullshit. I explain to my mother with a sense of urgency that I can't miss any more classes. She tries explaining that I'm in no shape to be in school, but it's like talking to a deaf man. Then my mother asks if I'd like something from the store. I don't respond.

She leaves the ward and comes back a short while later with the current issue of *Car and Driver*. Given my fondness for cars, maybe she thinks the magazine will quell my nerves. She hands it over and sits next to me on the bed. I stare at the cover and say to her, "Look at those headlights, they're getting messages from God."

I don't think this is quite the response my mother wanted. But in my mind I'm simply stating something of a factual nature, though the feeling of it is gone by now. It's no great revelation anymore. It's more along the lines of explaining the law of gravity, which is something my mother has a right to know.

A bit wiser from experience, my mother doesn't argue the matter one way or the other. She just sits next to me, trying to come up with comforting things to say. But I'm in no mood for motherly comfort. She senses this too, so she leaves the room and visits Terry to discuss my condition.

Camped out at the Heart of Auburn motel, my mother makes daily visits to the hospital, during which she sees Terry and me individually, and then all three of us meet for family sessions. These latter meetings are usually a battle where I plead my case to be discharged, and my mother and Terry join forces to squash my pleas. They do it in a courteous way, which makes it even tougher to take. I yell at both of them, accusing them of a conspiracy. Knowing how much my mother hates cussing, I deliver my tirades with every swear word I know. Then I note her conditioned response, which is mostly disgust and embarrassment.

Resorting to such tactics doesn't please me. I feel guilty for putting my mother through all this crap. I wish she would just give in to my demands and make it easier for both of us.

Our battle goes on for about four days, after which I realize that I'm not going to get my way. It's too much to handle — my mother, Terry, Dr. Jenkins and the nurses, all telling me how I'm not well and how I need to stay here in the hospital. With increasingly fragile nerves I give up the fight. In the back of my mind I'm hoping I can turn the tables when they least expect it, but for now the victory is theirs. The first casualty occurs when I agree to resign from classes for the winter quarter.

In exchange for cooperating, I'm allowed to go on supervised day trips outside the hospital with my mother who has control over the medication. While we're away she gets to decide whether I'm behaving appropriately and for how long I get to stay out. I feel like a dog on a leash. "Ready for a walk?"

"Ruff, ruff."

My mother and I have two outings together, each lasting the better part of a day. On our first excursion we do a fair amount of shopping, both at the mall and in downtown Auburn. My mother buys me a few cassette tapes of the music I want and some shirts and underwear. She had already made a trip on her own to CDV to get me some clothes and my Walkman, which is a true necessity in the mental ward.

The next thing on our agenda is to go to the parking lot of the Rus Uniform Company — the place where I camped out in my El Camino about 10 days ago, spellbound and entranced by my radio. It's here that I tossed my new watch out the car window, an action I now regret.

Maybe there's a chance we'll find it. We start by driving around the parking lot, relying on my memory for direction. When I sense we're getting warm, we park the car and commence combing the wooded area beyond the parking lot. My mother goes into the building to check with lost and found. Meanwhile, I scan around in expanding circles, neck bent to the ground. I'm like a tethered robot. My gait is stiff with an awkward shuffle, as if my vertebrae and joints were cemented on a stick. I can't fathom having the good fortune of finding my watch in a state such as this.

Feeling defeated, we leave without the watch and drive to Country's Barbecue for an early dinner. We never think to search for the watch with a metal detector. I don't think either of us has much in the way of brains today.

Opting for something a little more relaxing on the second outing, my mother and I drive down to Chewacla State Park for a hike and a much needed break from the sterility of the hospital. This might seem fun enough, but it ends up being far from it. With nine days worth of Loxitane built up in my system, I have to fend off an extreme case of grogginess. My movements are slow and my awkward gait is embarrassing. It's even worse than yesterday. Somehow I've also lost my endurance for the uphill climb. Normally I could run over three miles without much effort, and I've hiked in the Rockies above the timberline with good stamina. But now, in less than two weeks, I've turned into a character from *Night of the Living Dead*, trudging through the forests of East Alabama.

My mother tries to cheer me up. She says I'll get used to the medication, and maybe I won't need it for very long after all. I appreciate her efforts, but what does she know? No one's forcing this shit down her throat. The more we hike, the more frustrated I get, until finally we decide to turn back for the parking lot.

After an agitated dinner we're back at the hospital checking me in for the night. This is my mother's last day before driving to Atlanta and boarding a plane for Fort Lauderdale. She has a hard time fighting back the tears when she says goodbye. I give her a hug and tell her I love her. Then I walk back to my room with a flat numbness inside.

The psychiatric ward is quieter than usual. Neil is gone. My mother is back in Florida. None of the other patients are paying me any attention, and I don't care about them either. I turn my attention to the Walkman, going back and forth between my collection of cassettes and the local FM stations. I lie in bed for hours, not sleeping, just listening and hoping for a song that can transport my soul out of here.

Occasionally a good one comes on, bringing forth a sense of euphoria. It's a brief return to the way I felt in the El Camino sitting in the parking lot, and it feels like a gift from the heavens. The melody goes through me like a wave flowing through an otherwise flat surface. A single note separated by silence, then a voice picks up the harmony and I'm hanging on every word, carried to wherever the voice wants me to go. I wish it could last forever. But then the song comes to an end, taking the euphoria with it, and I'm back into a state of dullness.

It's the dull moments that are most common. At such times it doesn't matter what song is playing. It could be the very song that transported my soul the day before. Now it feels flat and lifeless and even irritating. So I shut it off and listen to nothing, but this is no better than the lousy song. Nothing can satisfy me. Everything sucks.

This is how I spend the idle hours in the psychiatric ward — lying in bed with headphones on, hoping for some kind of spiritual breakthrough, but mostly fending off the doldrums.

Two days after my mother's departure, my father and stepmother show up at the hospital. It's now Friday, February 3rd, and I've been here 12 days. I had a vague sense that my father was due to arrive, but I'm still surprised to see him in bodily form. He's on call everyday, ready to deliver a baby at a moment's notice. Unless he has a vacation planned months in advance, with full coverage from another doctor, he wouldn't be found out of beeper range. A sudden trip to Alabama is about as likely as an asteroid hitting the hospital.

What made him budge? I wonder. Then I remember an ordeal from earlier in the week. My mother and I were in a session with Terry—a comparatively calm session—until Terry said he called my father earlier in the day, asking him when he'd come up to see me. Apparently, my dad's reply was something like, "I'm pretty busy right now with my practice...so I don't know when I'll get the chance."

When Terry reported this back to my mother, she let all hell break loose. I've seen her angry before, but this went well beyond that. It might've been the last straw from years of conflict and a bitter divorce, or maybe she was overwrought with emotion over what was happening with me. It was probably a combination of both. Whatever the case, she was fuming mad and hardly responsive to Terry's calming efforts. All I can say is, it's a good thing Jenkins wasn't in the room because my mother might've been the recipient of a little Loxitane cocktail.

Eventually Terry was able to settle her down by agreeing to call my father again, this time with a greater sense of urgency. It was likely that second phone call that prompted my old man to make the trip.

He arrives while I'm sitting by myself in the day room. My headphones are on, but I take them off as soon as he approaches. We shake hands and walk down the hall to my room. It's late in the afternoon, but I'm still allowed a pass to leave the hospital with my dad until 9 P.M. My stepmother is waiting for us in the main lobby, and she gives me a hug when she sees me.

We get into the rental car and drive toward the Auburn campus. This is the first time my father's been up here, and I want him to be impressed. Sitting in the passenger seat, I navigate us down College Street, past Samford Hall with its ornate clock tower. Then we turn right onto Thatch Avenue, which takes us through the heart of campus. We drive by the library, then the Quad, then Haley Center and then past the football stadium on the right with the Coliseum to the left. I point out the CDV apartment complex, but we don't stop to go inside. It's time for supper, and I get to choose where we eat.

I pick a new restaurant on the Auburn-Opelika Highway called Po Folks, which specializes in home-style Southern cooking and cheap prices. I order the fried chicken dinner, including corn bread and your choice of two side items. The portions are huge, perfect for my appetite, and they come with free refills of sweet tea in mason jars. I have four or five refills of tea, thanks to the bone dry mouth that's still plaguing me. The tea is my anticholinergic salve, better than Cogentin.

It's a deeply satisfying meal for me, but my dad and step-mother don't seem all that impressed. I'm not convinced when they say their meals are fine, and I don't believe them when they make positive comments about the campus. Either I'm being too sensitive or they're a tough crowd.

The next morning my dad and stepmother arrive at the psychiatric ward to take me out for a full day pass. The head nurse tells me that this is my last day before being discharged tomorrow morning. She gives my father two capsules of Loxi-tane and a Cogentin tablet, which he's supposed to give me at the specified hours.

Once away from the hospital, I try convincing him that I really don't need the pills. My father nods in half-hearted agreement but doesn't say anything. It's not worth fighting over.

We drive through campus again, this time stopping at CDV to gather my stuff. It's a strange experience coming back here, kind of like recovering this other person from my past. I can't but help stare at my array of stuff: books, notebooks, cassette tapes, a calendar, photos, a cheap stereo system and clothing. Nothing looks out of the ordinary, except for the fact that my side of the room is immaculate. Everything is clean and order-ly, and all my clothes are washed and folded. Then I remember my mother. She was here while I was in the hospital, and she made my side of the room the pride of the entire apartment. Even Flash's side, which is normally the model of military order, looks a mess by comparison. It must be strange for Flash living here day after day. Everything was fine until mid-January. We would chat, play music, watch TV and drink beer on the weekends and then, *poof*, the roommate freaks out and vanishes. Now it looks like Flash is living with a well-tended museum display. The caption might read something like, *Here roomed an average college student, prior to his nervous breakdown.* Somehow, though, I can't quite picture it in the Smithsonian.

We pack my stuff into two large duffel bags, discarding what I consider junk, and we work as fast as we can before the roommates arrive. Once outside with bags in hand, we head to the car. There are students around watching us, me in particular, as we make our way to the parking lot. The last thing I want is to get into a talk about my recent experiences. The hospital, the drugs, the pleading with staff, the walking in on a guy masturbating in a bathtub—these aren't exactly things to be proud of. I avoid eye contact and say nothing.

Driving away, I consider seeing Phil to let him know I'm okay. But it's too late and the thought of it makes me sad. We're headed off campus for the last time. The sight of my El Camino in the parking lot might be the saddest thing of all.

Sensing my father and stepmother weren't pleased with last night's restaurant selection, I try to think of something more elegant. Auburn isn't known for elegance, so it's a bit of a stretch, especially in my state of mind. My creativity is plucked clean. To help the process along we stop by their motel room to consult the phone book. There's a listing for a restaurant in Opelika that was converted from an old mansion—someplace with the word *Tree* in it—and it sounds like a fine option.

After a quiet drive we pull up to the restaurant and almost

instantly I feel out of place. For one, I'm not dressed in the appropriate attire. I'm the only person in here wearing jeans and sneakers. The place is a far cry from your typical college hangout. It's decorated in Victorian style with the various rooms on the first floor serving as separate dining areas. Starched white linens are draped over the tables, which are topped with plum colored candles in pewter holders and flowers in glass vases.

The hostess guides us to a table somewhere off in a corner of one of the smaller rooms. Maybe she's trying to hide me from the other patrons. Once seated, I look at the menu and try to make sense of it. The room is so poorly lit that I can barely read the print. What I can see is a blurry mess of italicized nonsense, owing to the drugs, and the more I look at it the worse it gets until finally I give up and defer to my stepmother for an entrée selection. She's happy to help and she probably chooses something delicious, but I don't remember it. I just remember feeling awkward and stiff and out of place, like I'm wrapped in a cocoon of stupidity. I feel dumber than a pop-up toaster. I've got nothing to say about anything and no motivation to express the nothing I'm thinking. Somewhere in the shell that is my brain, I make a decision that I won't be recommending this restaurant in the future. I don't care how nice the fucking décor is.

9

THE following morning, as promised, I'm discharged from the East Alabama Medical Center. Part of the agreement is that I continue my treatment in Fort Lauderdale on an outpatient basis. I have one last visit with Dr. Jenkins. Then I'm on my way.

My Dad sits in on the last session during which he and Dr. Jenkins discuss my continuing treatment. First it's agreed that I'll be seeing a psychiatrist named Dr. Frei, my first appointment scheduled for tomorrow. Then the matter of my diagnosis is brought up.

Dr. Jenkins starts by rattling off the symptoms I had when I first came to the hospital and how these symptoms point to this or that diagnosis. He doesn't say the word *schizophrenia* outright, although you can tell that's what he's driving at. Instead, he gives me the diagnosis *Adjustment Reaction of Adolescence* because in his words it's the "less pejorative" label. He probably thinks I don't know what the word pejorative means, and he's right. I don't think my father knows either, but he doesn't ask for clarification. One fool is more than enough. Still I wonder, if all I have is a so-called adjustment reaction, then why do I have to take such strong medication?

Later I would understand the dilemma Dr. Jenkins faced. He knew that the label schizophrenia saddles the patient with the expectation that he'll be locked in a pattern of mental deterioration, maybe for life. Once the word gets attached to your chart you're in for hard-core drugs, and you're treated like a person afflicted with a serious brain disease, whether the diagnosis is valid or not. Even after the initial symptoms are gone and the drugs tapered off, the term *Schizophrenia—In Remission* is the typical diagnosis. The label is a sticky thing and, in the minds of most psychiatrists, you're never fully cured. This is why Jenkins defers to the lesser diagnosis.

But then why medicate me like a schizophrenic? According to the standard diagnostic manual, in order to accurately diagnose schizophrenia, the patient must show symptoms for at least six months. Yet psychiatrists and others in the mental health field often make the diagnosis after one short visit with a patient. Then they start up an immediate regime of neuroleptic drugs. It's right to question the ethics of administering these heavy hitting agents without an established diagnosis of schizophrenia, or some lesser psychotic affliction. But this is done routinely, often without probing much further than asking the question, "Are you hearing voices?" Answer "yes" and your prescription is as good as written.

I get the medication Loxitane, which is only approved for the treatment of psychotic disorders. Yet all I have, according to Dr. Jenkins, is an adjustment reaction. Maybe there's something fishy here and possibly unethical, but it's not unusual. Psychiatrists have been practicing this way for years. It's the philosophy of *First dope 'em up, then we'll see what we've got.* I get doped up, but what do we really have?

After my discharge session with Dr. Jenkins, I look around

the unit for Terry, but it's Sunday and he's not around. I want to hear him call me Big Guy one more time, and I want to tell him that he did a good job. It'll be a long time before I get the opportunity.

With my father driving and my stepmother in the back seat, we're headed to Atlanta, to the airport south of town. We'll be flying first class and I'm excited about it. It's my first time for such a luxury. Maybe my dad and stepmother want to spoil me. Or more likely, they're worried about me going psycho on the flight. Such an episode would be easier to contain in first class. Fortunately, there are no such outbursts to report.

Back in Fort Lauderdale, my dad drops me off at home where my mother is waiting for my arrival. She wants to make me something to eat, probably an egg sandwich or something, but I'm not hungry. She helps me unpack my stuff, and just like at CDV my old room is immaculate and ready for comfortable living. It doesn't seem like a place for a crazy person.

My sisters are home, and it's awkward being around them. The last time I talked with Julia was on the phone when I told her to watch MTV for messages from the Moon. This advice seems a little bizarre now, and I'm embarrassed to look at her. I feel the pressure of living up to her lofty image of me. For years she's looked up to me as her big brother. It's been annoying at times, like when she wore my shirts, usually my favorite ones, instead of her own. I've had to rummage through her closet to find them when they weren't on her. Her tendency to hang out with me and my friends got tiring as well. But it was also flattering to have the positive attention, knowing that I was important in her eyes. Now with my meltdown still fresh, I'm sure I've destroyed my favored status with her, and I don't stand a chance of getting it back.

It's a little easier talking with my older sister Christine, or at least it's less shame provoking. She's rebelled in the past, especially back in high school when she repeatedly took top honors on our mother's shit list. This makes Christine more approachable, and it's nice hearing her talk to me like I'm a normal guy. Even so, I can't take a lot of small talk right now, and I'm not willing to recount events over the past two weeks. So I extract myself from family chatter to unpack my belongings.

In our large ranch style home my bedroom is next to the family room and kitchen, just off the garage. The bedrooms of my mother and Julia are on the other side of the house beyond the living room. Christine lives in a small apartment in Pompano Beach with her boyfriend. Her old room is now a guest room where we keep rejected furniture.

My room served as a den for the previous owners, and it still has a den-like feel. The walls are paneled with the cheap brown stuff you find in mobile homes, and there's wall-to-wall carpeting the color of pea soup. I have an extra long twin bed so my feet don't hang over the end, which is the newest piece of furniture in the room. The remaining pieces have been here since kindergarten. They include a tall wooden bookcase — or étagère as my mother calls it — a desk and a dresser with two missing knobs. As a kid, I made a hobby of rearranging the furniture two or three times a year to make life a little more interesting.

There's a bathroom I consider my own, but you have to go through the family room to get to it. I used to imagine building a secret passageway, leading from my closet to the bathroom, so I wouldn't have to mess with the family room after showering. It's embarrassing when guests are over, and I have to walk through the family room with nothing on but a towel.

❀

Monday morning I have my first appointment with Dr. Rudy Frei. My mother takes time off from work to join me in our first session. Normally she'd be fulfilling her duties as a nurse conducting CAT scans and MRI's ordered by doctors.

We drive to the office on Commercial Boulevard, next to the fancy Raindancer restaurant. After a short wait Dr. Frei comes out to greet us. He's a tall lanky man with a peculiar Scandinavian accent. His face has a pressed-in look about it, but he carries himself in a stately manner, like royalty. Other than his height and unusual speech, the thing I notice right off about Dr. Frei is the way he dresses. He wears a wide assortment of colors—browns, oranges and deep reds seem to be his favorites—which is fine with me. But color coordination is not his shining talent. On this occasion he's wearing a green sport coat, like the kind you get when you win the Master's Tournament, with a light blue shirt and a brown dotted tie. I'm surprised his wife lets him out of the house that way.

Another trademark feature is the yellow legal pad he uses throughout our sessions, scrawling out copious notes as if words are of no value unless properly recorded. This feverish writing seems like a nervous habit—maybe a compulsion or a tic. Or maybe it's his excuse not to get into a lot of deep dialogue with his patients. "Hey I'm busy writing over here," he could say if pressed.

Our first session isn't anything special. It's mostly about my current mental status and plans for the future. Since I appear to be acting rationally without any delusions or hallucinations, he decides the medication is working and therefore maintains the Loxitane and Cogentin at the same levels. He also gives me a speech about my need to get into a regular routine while here in Fort Lauderdale, but this advice sounds suspicious, as though my mother put him up to it. I ask Dr. Frei how long he thinks I'll need to stay on the drugs.

"Let's wait and see how things progress," he says. The answer frustrates me to the point of anger, but I keep it in and try to look calm. I don't want him to know how I feel.

On the drive home I argue with my mother over the medication.

✻

The first few days back in Fort Lauderdale are mostly a blur. I don't feel ready to work for the moving company again, and all my friends are either working or away at college. My mother works full time, Julia's in school, and Christine's working at my stepmother's real estate office in Pompano Beach. This leaves me alone in the house all day with no car and nothing to do.

Most days I sleep in until 11 A.M. or so. Later, by 2 or 3 P.M., I'm exhausted again and craving a nap. If the weather is sunny, I nap outside on the lounge chair to get some color. My pattern is to lie in the sun for 15 to 20 minute intervals, between which I plunge into the pool to cool off.

At rare moments, when my laziness-induced guilt gets the upper hand, I'm driven to productive activity. One task is jogging the length of the neighborhood, which is a little over two miles. After that I might do some boxing in the garage, switching between the heavy bag and the speed bag. But this doesn't last very long. My rhythm is off and I get frustrated when the little bag spins out of control after an ill-timed punch. To calm my nerves I go inside and eat like a sedated pig.

My mother thinks she's helping to create a positive routine by giving me a list of chores to do each day. Typical entries include vacuuming the pool, cleaning the pool filter, sweeping out the garage, fixing the sprinkler by Julia's window and, with greatest frequency, cleaning my bathroom. I find these lists on the kitchen counter while pouring myself a bowl of cereal for breakfast. It irritates me to sit and ponder the dreaded list over my Golden Grahams. I don't know whether it's the content of the list or the fact that it's my mother ordering me around that I find so annoying—probably both. It's as if she's got me by the balls and won't let go until I do X and Y. Then the next day it's another list, with further testicular restraint, because it includes the unfinished items from the previous day.

She knows what I do and what I don't do, and she's keeping a running tally. There's no escaping it, except to actually do the things on the list. But with almost no energy and zero motivation, I provide the bare minimum of compliance.

The best I can hope for is the rare day when she's running late for work and has to go without leaving a list. On these days she usually calls from work around lunchtime to politely ask if I wouldn't mind doing the following chores.

10

AFTER about two weeks of this listless purgatorial crap, I decide it would be in my best interest to stop taking the medication. I don't tell Dr. Frei or anyone else about it, fearing I'll be hauled off to the nearest nuthouse.

A day or two after stopping the drugs, I notice more energy and better skill in putting my thoughts together. But I also start getting angry at my current situation. I decide that Dr. Frei doesn't have a clue as to how to handle my case, yet he has my parents convinced of his expertise.

Soon it's more than anger. I develop the power of mystical thoughts again. Now it's numbers rather than songs that have special significance. It could be anything from a serial number on an appliance to a phone number written on a note. Each number from one to nine has unique spiritual meaning, with zero representing the great void or the nothingness beyond the end of the universe. I interpret the sequence of numbers in a series as a message from the spirit world. This feels like a great revelation, and it's impossible to keep it to myself.

On February 22nd, the third day after stopping the drugs, I tell Dr. Frei about my numerical revelations. I tell him I'm doing fine, that this is best I've felt in weeks. But all he hears is that I stopped the drugs. He warns me of impending relapse and scares the bejesus out of me when he says I'll need to be hospitalized if I don't start taking them again at once.

At home after the session, I find the bottle of Loxitane and twist the cap off. I tap the bottle for a capsule to come out, but instead three come out, which seems significant. This must be a spiritual sign wherein three represents the Holy Trinity. So I take all three pills and repeat the process of tapping the bottle. Miraculously, three capsules come out again. I figure God wants me to take a certain number of pills, the effect of which will make me whole again. I go through this process a total of four times with three capsules coming out each trial. Now I've ingested the Holy Trinity four times, which is perfect because the number four represents completeness. After taking the 12 Loxitane capsules, a total of 600 milligrams, I put the cap back on and wait—for what, I'm not sure.

After dinner my mother notices that I'm not making a lot of sense, and I'm more groggy than usual. She asks if something's the matter. I decide it wouldn't hurt to tell her what I've done.

The story seems innocuous, hardly worth the look of concern on my mother's face. Before I finish explaining, she's up out of her chair dialing Dr. Frei. It's a quick conversation, after which my mother says we need to take a ride to the hospital. I think she's overreacting, as she's prone to do, but I'm too tired to argue. So I get in the car as requested.

Minutes later my mother and I are sitting in the emergency room area of the Imperial Point Medical Center, filling out forms and answering questions. This is the same hospital where Phil's mother died, and it's the same place where Phil nearly died of cancer. I'm not terribly thrilled to be here.

After an examination by the ER doctor, an attendant takes me up to the sixth floor, which is the mental ward. My mother rides the elevator with us but doesn't go onto the unit. She says goodbye in the hallway and tries to give me a hug, but I won't let her. Then a nurse escorts me to a room in the open part of the ward. One of the forms I signed downstairs must have been a voluntary admission agreement because otherwise I'd be in the locked unit. Checking the unlocked exit door confirms my hunch.

Within a few minutes of my arrival I bolt from the ward. Hobbling down the staircase, I reach the second floor, but that's all. Some kind of code is announced over the PA system, and in a matter of seconds I'm surrounded by security guards. I board the elevator without resistance. Guards are at my side as we ascend back to the sixth floor. Now I'm assigned a room in the locked section.

One of the social workers shows me around the place to get me oriented. He asks me to relinquish any valuables in my possession, including my wallet and the new watch my father bought me after I tossed the first one. I refuse to give up these things, insisting that I'll be released from the hospital tomorrow. "My stuff is safer with me anyway," I say.

I sleep through the night and get up earlier than usual. After breakfast, I wait in the small lounge to be discharged. I'm exercising great self-control by waiting with such calm. Soon there should be a person with a key who'll unlock the door and let me out of here. It should be clear to all that my being here is a silly misunderstanding.

For about two hours I play the patient waiting game, which to me is plenty of time. I finally ask the nurse about getting out, and she defers the question to Dr. Frei who, conveniently, isn't on the floor. Next, I ask her for my Walkman, which I know is around here somewhere. It's one of the few essential items I thought to bring. Again the nurse defers to Dr. Frei who apparently wrote a note in my chart stating that I'm not allowed to have it at this time. So now I'm zero for two and not too happy about it.

I demand to know why I can't listen to my own goddamn radio. But the nurse ignores me, saying only that she won't talk to me while I'm using such an abrasive tone. A surge of anger rises inside me, signaling the end of my patient waiting game. I start telling other patients that they shouldn't put up with this crap. I tell an elderly woman that the medication she just took will make her sick, and she should vomit it out if she has any sense left.

The no-nonsense nurse calls for help from the male staff, and they arrive swiftly like a pack of rugby players. The most muscular of the bunch pats me on the shoulder. He's a good natured guy who tries to turn the whole thing into a comedy. I like his attitude, so I follow him when he asks me to join him in the seclusion room. It's the oldest trick in the book, and I'm falling for it.

Unbeknownst to me, there's a nurse situated by my ass with a syringe. She says it'll do me some good. Without much of a fight, I let her poke me with the thing. Now I'm the recipient of five milligrams of Haldol.

Mission accomplished, the staff leaves the room while the nurse locks the door behind her. I'm supposed to settle down, and I actually do for a while. I sit at the end of the bed, getting up at intervals to pace around the room. Then I lie on the bed trying to make sense of the plaster marks on the ceiling.

After about two hours in seclusion Dr. Frei arrives to check on me. His familiar face brightens me up. I figure he's here to give me a little lecture and then let me go home. We talk about the overdose and what this means as far as my mental stability is concerned. Feeling less sure of myself, I try to explain it away, taking pains not to mention God's part in the overdose or the mystical significance of the numbers. But I probably slip up in this regard because Dr. Frei tells me that I'll need to stay in the hospital for a while, until I'm stabilized. He adds that I'm not ready to leave the seclusion room.

I plead my case with renewed urgency, knowing he's about to leave. But except to say that I'm "not well," Dr. Frei ignores me. This makes me want to hit him, but I don't. Instead, when he goes to leave, I hold him up by blocking the doorway. I tell him I don't like being ignored and I won't let him leave without hearing me out.

He signals through the door's small Plexiglas window for staff to help him out, saying he'll see me tomorrow after I've calmed down. I lunge toward the door, but one of the orderlies is there to push me back. I'm no match for him today. While backpedaling I can hear the sound of the deadbolt.

I'm alone in the tiny room again but not as calm this time. I kick the door and hurl out a barrage of profanity at top volume. Minutes later, a nurse and a group of male staff come in to give me another shot of Haldol. I refuse it this time, figuring that I'll get an opportunity to argue the matter through. But there's no debate. The nurse backs away while the attendants wrestle me down nose-first to the bed. Then they flip me over so I'm lying on my back. I see leather cuffs and straps coming toward me.

As they're strapping me down to the bed, they take pains to be courteous about what they're doing, which is comforting and sinister at the same time. The most annoying part is their habit of repeating my name as they explain the process. The ringleader says, "Okay Brett, we're putting a cuff around your left ankle." Then he asks, "Brett is that too tight?"

A process of negotiation develops among the staff about the right amount of tension for the cuff—somewhere between "too tight" and "I think he could get out of that." Once they get it to the right tension, they insert a leather strap through the

metal ring on the cuff and secure the other end of the strap to
the steel bed frame. One man works the cuffs and straps, while
the others hold me down until there's a secure cuff attached
to both wrists and both ankles. These are called four-point restraints or two-by-two restraints, if you want to be technical.

When I'm sufficiently staked down to the bed, I have the
ability to move my limbs about six inches from side to side.
Any more than that and it's considered too loose. An itch on
the scalp is a small dose of hell. Now under firm control, I'm
no match for the needle. The nurse says it'll be a lot better
for me if I relax while receiving the shot, as if that's the natural thing to do. Then she gives me a shot of Haldol, followed
by something new—7.5 grams of sodium amytal, which she
says is "for agitation." The effect is almost instantaneous. I'm
asleep and snoring for the better part of the afternoon.

After my involuntary nap, I wake up mad and loud, which
gets the attention of another needle-wielding nurse. Again I
get shots of Haldol and sodium amytal, and once again I'm
thrust into sleep.

I wake up for dinner feeling hungry, but I wonder how the
hell I'm supposed to eat all strapped down like this. One of
the attendants comes in and releases my left wrist to accommodate me. I guess he figures, since I'm right handed, my left
would be the weaker limb. He'll take his chances with the left
jab over the right hook. Fortunately for both of us, I'm not in
a fighting mood. I fumble with the food and try to carry on a
conversation with the guy at the same time.

I'm having troubling thoughts that I share with the orderly.
I tell him about this worldwide conspiracy underway to destroy freethinking people. I don't tell him my life is in jeop-
ardy, figuring that I'll be able to outsmart the conspiratorial
forces. Instead, I warn the attendant that he's in serious danger.
I explain that he won't be able to recognize it at first, but there

are clones and robots walking around disguised as human beings.

The man gives me a concerned nod.

After mealtime, I'm rewarded for my good behavior with
the removal of one of the ankle cuffs. So now my right leg and
left arm are at liberty to move about the bed. What will I do
with these new freedoms? The most urgent task is urination,
but the staff won't let me go to the bathroom. Instead, a nurse
comes in to give me a plastic urinal and then she leaves so I
can do my business in private.

It's an awkward task pissing sideways in bed with your
non-dominant hand, which has to simultaneously aim and
keep the urinal from spilling. Meanwhile, there's the constant
monitoring through the window in the door. I'm almost afraid
that someone will come up to the window and say "Boo!" in
the midst of my stream. Despite all this, I get the job done
without incident.

In two-point restraints, I sleep in the seclusion room
throughout the night. At scheduled intervals a staff person
comes in to take my blood pressure and check the movement
of my limbs. Shortly before breakfast the attendants remove
the restraints, but I still have to stay in seclusion.

This pisses me off. About an hour after breakfast I start
asking from my bed to be let out of here.

No one seems to hear me. Maybe their plan is to ignore
me. So I talk louder, demanding immediate release.

Still no answer.

More enraged, I get out of bed and pound the door with
closed fists. I think of the most abusive things to say, and I yell
them while pounding and kicking the door.

If it were only attention I want, my wish would be granted. Just like the day before, I'm wrestled down by a group of
leather-wielding men who grab hold of my limbs and repeat
the process of putting me in four-point restraints. It takes a

little longer this time for the staff to go about their business due to my kicking and trying to land punches. Each of my four limbs has a man stationed there ready for my assaults. I commence spitting, but my mouth is all dry and the spit goes nowhere. Their defense is to drape a towel over my head.

I wish above all for superhuman strength. How great it would be if I could break free of the straps, reach up with arms extended, grab an attendant's head in each hand and smash them together like exploding grapefruit. But then the reality of the situation sinks in. I'm fully restrained and shot up with a heavy dose of sodium amytal.

A rock-hard sleep follows immediately.

Dr. Frei arrives late in the morning accompanied by two of the male staff for protection. I have to be roused out of a dead sleep and I can't shake the grogginess. Slurring my words, I tell Dr. Frei that I want out of here. But he doesn't seem to hear me. He's out of the room in no more than a couple of minutes.

At the nurse's station Dr. Frei makes a change in my medication. Given the extent of my hostility, he decides to try me on a different medication—one with more sedating side effects. His choice is Thorazine, 200 milligrams, four times per day. He continues the Cogentin to help combat Thorazine's side effects and he keeps an order for sodium amytal, as needed, in case I need a knockout punch.

The day is a waste. I'm either sleeping or lying silent in a state of groggy oblivion. At 4 P.M. the staff awards me the privilege of three-point restraints. And, by seven, they take me down to the familiar two points. As a further bonus, since I'm nearly comatose, they decide to hold off my medication until some degree of vitality returns.

By 10 P.M. I feel somewhat rejuvenated. Again I ask to be released from seclusion, but there's no answer. So again I yell out, demanding my release. By this time I sort of know my wish won't be granted. I'm no genius, but I understand this tiring sequence and its outcome.

Something new is called for to break the pattern. The thing I come up with is to urinate on the floor. This will turn the tables, I think. But all it gets me is an upgrade back to three-point restraints with only my left arm free to move about.

A short while later, one of the male orderlies comes in to clean up the mess. I try the strategy of friendliness with him. I also let him know that I still have to use the bathroom. "Number two," I say.

He arranges for me to be escorted out of seclusion so I can toilet myself and stretch my limbs. On the trip back to the seclusion room, I plead with the charge nurse not to make me go back in there, begging for human decency. But the answer from her is "not yet."

Newly infuriated, I hurl my body around to land a punch on the guy to my left. But the element of surprise is missing. The punch is all air. Then I get jerked to the floor belly-flop-style, and I'm dragged back to the familiar bed with its full assemblage of four-point restraints. A fresh injection of sodium amytal in the ass completes the encounter.

That should've done the trick to put me to sleep, but I've been sleeping all day. Instead I lie in bed agitated, yelling at the night staff, slurring my words. It's a shining moment for mankind.

On the third day of seclusion I become more manageable. It's sinking in that the yelling and the combativeness aren't getting me what I want, and I don't want this room to be my permanent address. I put on a pleasant manner and don't say anything about getting out of here. Maybe they'll let me out if they think I like this place.

By 9 A.M. I'm down to two-point restraints, and shortly

after lunch I'm released from the cuffs and straps and free to move about the locked room.

A couple of hours later Dr. Frei arrives for his daily checkup. I try to keep things pleasant, but it's hard to ignore the fact that my speech is a garbled mess. Dr. Frei acknowledges the obvious, that it's due to the drugs, and he assures me it will pass. Then he saves the day by authorizing my release from solitary confinement. Maybe he's not so bad after all.

But this thought passes quickly once I realize his intention is to put me in two-point restraints in a regular bed with the side rails up. The only difference between this room and seclusion is a window with a view. The room is spacious and bright, but cuffed to a bed I can't make much use of it. If there was another patient in the room before, he's gone now. The door is kept wide open, and an assigned staff person drops by to observe me every 10 minutes or so.

Looking out the window almost makes the situation feel worse than before. I can see fluffy clouds drifting across the blueness of the sky, and if I crane my neck I can see the flat expanse of metropolitan Fort Lauderdale. Palm trees wave in the breeze while distant office buildings reflect the glare of the sun. I see roofs of houses and streets with cars driving around. Everything seems alive and content down there. I think of the people driving from place to place and how they've all got their shit together. I wonder what the hell I'm doing in here anyway. The thought gets me sort of worked up again, which leads me to call out and ask, as politely as I can muster, to be released from the hospital.

By this time the staff must be as frustrated with me as I am with them. They don't want me back in seclusion, but they can't tolerate another episode. So the head nurse comes into my room and explains the situation as best she can. She then offers me the only solution at her disposal—an injection of sodium amytal. Dutifully, I reveal a suitable patch of skin. And once again, I'm thrust back into unconsciousness.

The sleep lasts about three hours after which I wake up groggy and confused and with a full bladder. I can barely walk as I'm escorted to the bathroom. My legs are like Jell-O, and I feel like I'm about to faint.

With luck, I make it to the bathroom and back. Upon returning to bed, I ask if I could please go without the restraints, telling the nurse that I'll feel a lot more comfortable that way.

By now I'm used to having my requests denied, no matter how pleasantly I state them. This time the nurse tells me that the restraints and rails must remain in place for my own protection. Due to the high level of medication, I'm at risk for falling out of bed.

How can I argue with such reasoning? Since I can't, I shut up and sleep with the two-point restraints.

Early the next morning I'm at last granted freedom from the cuffs and straps.

11

I F this is a battle of wills, then surely the staff led by Dr.
Frei is winning and I'm losing. I'm like a beaten dog that
cowers whenever a hand is raised near its face, or like
one of the robots I was warning the orderly about. On my first
day out of seclusion, I sit in the small lounge and stare at the
floor without saying much of anything. If I talk my voice is
a monotonous drone, and if asked a question I give a brief
monosyllabic response. The most emotion you can get out of
me is a sigh.

I've developed this peculiar habit of wringing my hands.
It's like I'm trying to shake off the nerves or shake the monkey
off my back, but my thoughts aren't clear enough to make a
connection. The hand wringing is only one of the many side
effects of the medication. To Dr. Frei it's a worthwhile trade-
off. But I think that if you weren't crazy before, you'll certainly look the part when the drugs take over.

This robotic state is the way I feel most of the time, as
if my brain were wiped clean, like a computer purged of all
memory except for the basic operating system. I can eat, sleep,

walk and toilet myself, but not much more than that. Ask me the name of the president and I'll give you a blank stare.

Then there are rare moments when my thoughts seem to go all over the place, without clear boundaries separating one from another. In psychiatric jargon it's known as *loose associations*, but the term does little justice to the experience. It's a flurry of ideas coming at me, like the visual sensation of driving at night through a snowstorm with the high beams on. Hundreds of thoughts fly by, each one clamoring for attention. To the outsider, it doesn't look like very much is going on. A typical entry in the patient's chart might read: *Patient sitting quietly in day room with good behavioral control.* But engage the patient in conversation and it's a different story. The new chart entry would read something like: *Patient is exhibiting a flight of ideas and magical thinking*, which describes both the process and the content of the thoughts. In psychiatric language this would be considered a full account of what's going on. To experience this state is another matter, one that can't be summed up by pet phrases. It's like being in the nexus of thought, feeling and sensation, where the world is fully alive. And it feels like being reunited with primitive life, before the advent of concepts and classifications.

At times such as this I'm compelled to share my thoughts with others, which makes me come off wackier than usual. There's this pressurized quality to my voice, like I'll explode if I don't get it all out. My target audience is the other patients who don't give me the same tired lines about how I'm not well and how I need to get stabilized. I want human contact that isn't pre-packaged. And I want everyone to agree with my way of thinking. The feeling is almost overpowering. I'm here to save the world through the philosophy of liberation from brainwashing, and I'll fight for freedom to the end!

Or so it seems for the moment.

Beneath the preaching, I can feel a sense of being on shaky

ground, like I've entered the territory of the fanatic, trying to convert the world. It's an inner sense of doubt that mocks my every word. I fend it off with what I think are stronger and more compelling arguments, which work for a while.

It's been said that the flip side of fanaticism is doubt. This rings true for me because in order to be a fanatic you have to fend off a lot of competing information. Anything not in harmony with your philosophy is a threat, including tangible evidence to the contrary.

Still, it's amazing how long people can remain wrapped in their fanaticism. Years and years are spent trying to convert others while fending off doubts. Fundamentalist Christians are prime examples of this. They don't know it, but they're hammering you with doubt-riddled ideas. They use a hammer called religious faith, with the doctrine of God and Jesus embedded in the message. But inside the hammer is doubt. Their defensiveness around groups that believe differently makes the point. It would be a frightening thing to open up the hammer and look earnestly at their insecurity, at their doubt. I wouldn't want to face it. It's a lot easier knocking people in the head repeating, "Have you accepted Jesus Christ as your personal savior?"

I have a hammer too, but it isn't quite the same. My hammer doesn't have the authority of the Church or the endorsement of any organization behind it. I'm alone, swinging away in a locked ward, filled with doubt, but not looking at it, trying to save souls. It's a precarious place to be.

Wielding a doubt-riddled hammer isn't limited to mental patients or religious fanatics. While I hammer away with my unusual ideas, Dr. Frei employs his own version of the hammer on me. Just as fundamentalist nuts are endorsed by the power of organized religion, Dr. Frei has the backing of mainstream psychiatry in his corner. The doctrine in this case is the biochemical disease model of human suffering. It's a simple theory that reduces the broad range of human miseries—aberrant thoughts, depression, compulsive behaviors and so on—down to biology. Biochemistry is destiny. Biochemistry is akin to God.

Within this framework, the psychiatrist's job is to treat the symptoms with an appropriate chemical weapon. This usually means drugs, although electric shock may be used for depression, and frontal lobotomies were used in the not-so-distant past. In fact the hammer used on me, Thorazine, is the same drug that revolutionized psychiatry in the 1950's, replacing the frontal lobotomy as a treatment of choice for psychosis.

Thorazine is like a lobotomy in a pill, and it's a biochemical hammer if ever there was one. It does what a hammer is supposed to do. It whacks the brain, knocking out the problem symptoms while also shutting down the part of the mind that is responsible for creativity, spontaneity and higher reasoning. These so-called side effects turn the patient into a leaden zombie. But that's okay. After all, the doctor says the most important thing is to eradicate the psychotic symptoms. No worry that the patient has turned into a vegetable—a hammerhead. That's part of the deal. There's no free lunch.

Does it matter that the patient underwent some kind of trauma prior to the onset of the symptoms? What about family crises? Does any of this matter to mainstream psychiatrists? For most, the answer is no because it doesn't change the treatment approach. Those troubling events might have pushed the patient over the edge, but the real battleground is biology. Past events don't fit into this treatment model, so it's a waste of time pursuing them.

Imagine a carpenter with nothing but a hammer. With no other tools at his disposal, his job is to tear down an old house and build another in its place. He might fare okay on destroying the old house, smashing down walls and such. But I doubt he'd get very far trying to build a new house with nothing but a hammer. In fact, it's impossible. He hasn't learned about the miter saw, the drill, electrical wiring, gas lines, plumbing or duct work. All he knows is the hammer. To me, this sums up the problems inherent in modern, mainstream psychiatry. They know how to go into your brain and hammer away at your biochemistry. But what about repairing the cracks in your self-concept or exploring the longings of your injured soul? Unless you can fit these into a 15 minute session, forget about it.

On my fourth day of being hospitalized, I'm considered stable enough to have family visitors. My mother arrives first but stays less than a half-hour. I'm mad at her for bringing me here, and I can't stand hearing her side of the story. If I express how angry I am I'll look like a raging lunatic, thus risking another stay in the seclusion room. That's the last place I want to go.

I feel damned either way. If I show what I'm really feeling, they'll lock me up in four-point restraints. If I'm obedient, they've won another battle. To stay out of trouble I keep everything inside, especially with the staff. I say only shallow pleasantries or I don't say anything.

It's easier talking with the other patients, especially the elderly, who aren't as judgmental for some reason. As such, they're the best people for testing out ideas and building confidence. Occasionally I let out a profane word, like "shit" or "goddamn" when making my point, which always gets the staff on alert. One of the nurses tells me I have a good vocabulary, so why do I have to use such language? She reminds me of my mother, who once washed my mouth out with Dial soap when I was about 12. She resorted to this after I let out a particularly bad barrage of profanity. The taste of the soap was horrible, and I coughed and spat all over the sink. It was unforgettable punishment, but it did little to curb my language, except possibly around my mother.

Now in my defense I tell the nurse that watering down your language is like living in bondage. In return, she gives me a little civics lesson on the virtues of respecting others' sensibilities. I listen like a good patient, but I doubt the speech will be any more effective than my mother's Dial soap.

After dinner I refuse my last dose of Thorazine for the day, saying that it's a free country and I don't need drugs anyway. But the point isn't up for debate. My options are to take the drug orally or by injection, with or without the use of restraints, depending on whether I put up a struggle. With my reasoning somewhat intact, I take the goddamn drug orally with clenched fists.

I call my mother later in the evening to vent my frustration. She's the best audience for such purposes, even though I'm still angry with her. While we're talking I let down my armor for a few minutes and start sobbing out of self-pity. I'm plagued by the eternal question, "Why me?"

The tears dry up when I notice one of the social workers looking at me.

After the call I go over to play backgammon with one of the male patients who's about my age, but I can't concentrate on the game. The guy leaves out some of the rules, and I don't know how to play the game anyway. I feel frustrated and angry, but like the tears I have to shut that down too. The seclusion room is only a few feet away and I can feel myself flirting with it. I'm a flood of emotion with grief and anger simmering just below the surface. Numbness is my only alternative. It's the safest thing. But under the numbness, I'm like molten lava.

12

I T takes a lot of energy and a lot of Thorazine, but I persist in my compliance for two more days and I'm rewarded for it. On the 29th of February, leap year day, I'm transferred next door to the open psychiatric ward.

Things are livelier here, with more people and more activities to replace the hours of boredom. At first I'm reluctant to get involved. It feels safer to spend my waking hours staring out the window at the sky and the South Florida landscape. The view seems more impressive than from the locked side.

Looking westward I notice a familiar sight. It's the home of Charley, an ex-boyfriend of my older sister Christine. I always liked him, and I had hoped he and my sister would stay together. While they were dating a couple of years ago, he was flying small airplanes, working his way up to being an airline pilot. I flew with him once in a little rented Cessna. We did touch-and-go landings, and Charley had the tiny aircraft upside down for about 15 seconds. Then he let me steer the plane, but I was feeling nauseous and disoriented, and I didn't enjoy it.

Far more enjoyable was the time when Charley, his friend Don and Christine and I took a road trip up to Disney World in the summer of '82. We traveled in Charley's parents' Winnebago and drank beer almost nonstop throughout the trip. Don was a close friend of Charley's, but the two of them were like night and day. Charley was even tempered and polite, almost to a fault, while Don was about the crudest guy you'd ever hope to meet. He was the kind of guy who farted while driving, then locked the windows shut so you couldn't get any relief. For him every other word was *shit* or *fuck*, and when he used longer words, like ones with four syllables, he'd blend in the F-word for added effect. Like if the Miami Dolphins won last Sunday, to him they didn't just win, they reigned *vicfuckingtorious*. If Don were living in my house, my mother wouldn't be able to stock enough Dial soap.

For added pleasure on our trip Don brought along a little bottle of white powder, and he showed me how to snort the stuff. This was scary to me, but I did it anyway. I had tried marijuana and didn't think much of it, but this was a lot more risky. The snort produced a cold mentholated surge and then a nosebleed, which soon went away.

In a matter of seconds I was propelled into a state of manic euphoria. I now knew what Sigmund Freud must've felt like. But instead of analyzing dreams or poking and prodding into patients' sexual fantasies, I was frolicking in the land of Mickey Mouse and Donald Duck. I remember riding the roller coaster *Space Mountain* with a locked grin, interrupted only by hysterical laughter. We repeated the ride three or four times with the same ecstatic result.

After being under the seductive spell of cocaine on that trip, I vowed never to do it again. For the sake of accuracy, I should mention that I broke the vow once in '83 while partying with friends in Gainesville—a little escapade resulting in a coed skinny-dipping party at 4 A.M. The next day I was wiped out, with bloody scabs in my nose. Not that I wanted to become a saint or anything, but that wasn't exactly how I wanted to conduct my life.

So now I'm sitting here in the day room, gazing out the window at Charley's house with the familiar Winnebago parked alongside, half on the grass. It's like looking at freedom itself. Reckless as our trip was, it was still freedom, and that's what I'm aiming for.

"What are you looking at?" one of the elderly patients asks. He has a friendly face that sags in the right places. So I tell him the story of Charley's Winnebago and the Disney trip with my sister and Don's crazy powder. I get it all out, and I think the old man understands what I'm saying—not just the words but also the longing behind the words.

After telling the story, I feel closer to this old man than anyone else in the place. I think maybe now I have a friend. His name is Arthur and he's about 70 or so, tall and overweight with white hair and a reddish face. He's a shaky, nervous man with demons inside, but I can tell he won't do me any harm.

A day or so later, I start getting more involved in the activities of the unit, trying to fight off the boredom any way I can. There are group therapy sessions, arts and crafts groups and games. Occasionally, we go down for a chaperoned walk onto the hospital grounds for fresh air. This is something they call *recreational therapy*, which I suppose sounds good to health insurance companies, better than the reality of standing out on the grass like zombie lawn ornaments. On rare occasions I go down to the exercise room on the ground floor, but only when there's extra staff available to watch me. More often, I play Ping-Pong with the other patients and staff.

I feel like a clumsy oaf at the Ping-Pong table, but still manage to beat nearly everyone I play, which isn't saying much. There's this one social worker named Larry who probably lets me win to help build my fragile self-esteem. I accuse him of this, but he denies it, saying that I'm a "born athlete." I've never been told such a thing before, nor do I believe him, but it sounds good hearing it anyway. Truth be told, Larry is more of a born athlete than I'll ever be, with his stocky build and his wealth of knowledge about sports and fitness. He gives me workout advice down in the gym and dietary tips at mealtime, as if he's training me for my next big bout with the champion.

One piece of advice he gives me is that you should eat your meal to completion before consuming any beverage. This way your digestive system works more efficiently, and you'll have more energy. I notice that Larry eats his own meals like this, so at least there's consistency between his words and actions. In this small way he seems like a man of integrity, someone I could possibly trust.

The second day on the open ward, Larry tells me I need a shave. I'm looking pretty grisly by this time, having gone three or four days in the locked unit without shaving. He gives me what looks like a generic hospital-issue razor and a tiny packet of shaving cream. He mentions something about how I'll be more approachable to the women if I have a clean-shaven face, which to me is a meaningful incentive. Larry has a knack for enlisting one's motivation.

So I commence shaving my long stubble with the razor. It's a pathetic instrument for the task at hand, and soon I'm cursing at the blood and the nicks and the ineffectiveness of the whole operation. I think I'd make more progress with a butter knife. This cheap piece of shit razor is pissing me off, and I can't stand it! I twist the thing into a pretzel and toss it into the toilet. Then, after my shower, I sit in the day room to cool off.

Larry comes over and asks me where the razor is. I remember the speech about how you're not allowed to have any so-called *sharps* in your possession, "for your own safety and for the safety of others." How you could kill anyone with that little shit on a stick is beyond me, but I don't want to start anything.

"I put it in the toilet bowl," I tell him, as if that's the natural thing to do.

He looks at me hard for a moment. Then he goes to find rubber gloves so he can retrieve the damn thing out of the commode. I feel like a shameful moron all over again.

The next day he brings me a decent twin-blade razor, and it works pretty well. At least Larry won't have to go dredging for it.

Now that I'm more approachable to the staff, we're able to talk about some of the things going on in my life. We spend most of our time discussing my family, especially my father and the role he might have played in my illness. It's the first time I've thought about my dad this way. Up to now, it's been just a series of quick reactions and impressions with no coherence. I might've felt mad at him for some sarcastic remark he made, or grateful after he did something nice for me, but once the feelings passed I let it go. I've always wanted my father to like me, and I think maybe he does, but he has his own way of showing it. That's as far as I've ever explored the situation.

But now, in group therapy, I'm supposed to delve into what it was really like all these years with him as a father, and I discover that I have a captive audience. Talk about my old man and the staff hangs on my every word. To the therapists, the more I discuss him, the more I'm growing and gaining that all important quality *insight*. But I don't think it's the happy memories they want to hear about. They want the dirt and the motivations behind the dirt. This doesn't take a lot of searching. Some of the questions that come up are, "Why did your father leave your mother for another woman?" "When was the last time he gave you a hug?" "Why did he miss your high school graduation?" And, "why is he emotionally unavailable when he visits?" These turn into high priority topics among the social work staff.

The momentum of the group leads to the topic of my parents' divorce and how I first found out they were splitting up. I tell the story without reluctance.

I was seven years old. My mother was sitting on one of the chairs out back near the pool with tears in her eyes. My dad stood away from her not saying much of anything. Soon I knew they were talking about me.

"You've got to tell him. It's your responsibility," I could hear my mother saying.

My dad agreed but didn't come over to me right away. Instead, he talked with my mother a few more minutes while I waited for him on the couch in the family room. My sisters must've been somewhere else that day.

Soon enough, there was my father giving me the stiff speech about how he wasn't going to be living here with us anymore. He said we'd see each other on regular visits and how that would be lots of fun. He looked concerned as he said all this, and he gave me a friendly pat on the knee. I didn't move or say anything.

Later, when I saw my mother crying, I cried too. I was sad but mostly I was scared for what would happen from now on. I was afraid we would have to move from the neighborhood and that I'd never see dad or Phil again. Maybe the family wouldn't be able to survive with just my mom at the helm. My father was leaving, I was just a weak boy, and my mother didn't exactly seem like a pillar of stability. There was a sense of impending doom.

As I wrap up the story, fending off tears, I can see that the group is focused squarely on me, and I'm getting more attention and more sympathy than I expected. Soon my father earns the designation of being neglectful, and I'm the helpless victim. The support of the group feels real, and it's good to get this stuff out. But what am I supposed to do now?

At first I think maybe this is enough. Just complain about my dad, get lots of support and sympathy, feel vindicated and then—*presto*—wounds are healed. But there's something bothering me. While holding up the neglectful father image, I shut out the good things about him. I forget about him supporting us financially all these years and how, even though he was sometimes late picking us up, he never once missed a visit.

There was one time when my father nearly beat up the manager of a bowling alley for yelling at me after I walked up one of the lanes. I remember him saying, "Don't you ever talk to my son that way!" He was ready to fight for me.

But this type of anecdote doesn't fit with the image we're creating at Imperial Point, so I dismiss it. I also dispel my father's lessons on how to repair cars, how to install stereo systems and how to properly use the all important power tools in his garage. I shut out the times he showed up for my football games and took pictures of me from the bleachers like a lot of other proud fathers did. My old man and I had some good talks too, which were some of the best moments I had with him. But they don't mean anything now. I want to feel vindicated as the neglected son, and the therapists are allies helping the cause.

One such ally, a skinny male social worker whose name I can't remember, comes into my room and asks questions about my family. Sometimes he sits at the foot of my bed while I'm sitting up in it. His soft voice is strangely familiar, but I can't place it.

After a few of these room service counseling sessions, the guy starts to give me the creeps. One day we're talking about my father, and I start filling up with emotion. The social worker reaches over and starts rubbing my shoulder, saying that it's okay if I feel like crying.

Right away my guard goes up. "Fuck you, I ain't crying for you!" I think to myself, but don't say anything. He must sense my discomfort because right after my freeze up he leaves the room.

After he's gone, I have to talk with someone about the creepiness. Arthur is the person I look for, and I find him reading the Sun-Sentinel in the day room. He tells me that the social worker is gay and that I'm pretty ignorant if I can't see it for myself. With that, I feel the full brunt of my stupidity.

After the lights are off for bedtime, I lay awake tossing and battling with the sheets until the small hours of the morning. When I finally do sleep, I have a kind of hellish homosexual nightmare. In the dream I'm cuffed to a cinder block wall in what seems like a dungeon and I'm forced to watch men getting it on with other men. The gay social worker puts a cuff on my ankle. I spit at him to shoo him away, but I'm weak and can't stop him from cuffing me and ripping at my clothes. I wake up panic stricken only to fall asleep to another nightmare as graphic as the first.

By morning I'm a mess, wandering the halls and wondering what the hell the dreams mean. I think I'd rather die than live out what I saw in those dreams. While dreaming, I was powerless to do anything. But in real life I could kill myself rather than being subjected to such torture.

The idea seems to help. At least now I have a sense of control back. The next thing is to tell the social worker that he's not welcome back in my room. I work over the lines in my head and get a pretty clear idea what to say.

There's something else going on in my head as I try to figure all this out. It's a series of disturbing memories from elementary school. I haven't thought about this stuff for years, but now it's back at full strength. And now I can remember why the episode with the social worker felt so eerily familiar. His voice is the same, or nearly the same, as my old grade

school teacher Mr. Bowen. He was my teacher at Christ Methodist School from first grade until the middle of fourth when
he was fired for sexual misconduct.

The first year or so I thought he was a great teacher, like an
older pal or a new dad. He was kind and playful, always there
to help with any problem you had. He acted fatherly, but he
was more carefree than your average dad. Learning was a joy
back then, mostly because of Mr. Bowen's ability to bring the
subject matter to life.

We had these annual class trips that everyone got excited
about. One was a trip to Kentucky to go spelunking in Mammoth Cave. There was great anticipation as we marked off the
days on the calendar before departing. To prepare for the trip,
we studied the geology of the cave and the people who explored it. We learned about stalactites and stalagmites, and we
learned about these strange blind fish swimming in underwater
lakes, and about this guy named Floyd who got stuck in a narrow passage for weeks in the 1930's before dying despite a
number of failed rescue attempts. What a thrill to go exploring
in such a mysterious place! The trip proved to be one of the
best events of my early school years. It stands in stark contrast
to the horror of Mr. Bowen's darker side.

At first he didn't bother me, and I don't think he did much
to the other boys either. At least I didn't notice anything going on. But midway through the second grade things started to
change. There was the day he was supposed to get urine samples from all the kids for some kind of physical or something.
I think the girls were allowed to pee in privacy, but he had all
us boys line up naked while he sat there with little plastic cups
in his hand. I was suspicious of this being wrong somehow but
didn't say anything about it.

Then there were times he had us boys run around the room
naked, chasing each other while he observed. And on the annual trips he watched us in the bathtub, reminding us to wash

our private parts *real good.*

There were two or three times during recess when Mr. Bowen came over to me alone and had me pull my pants down part of the way. Then he asked me these strange questions, like whether I ever played around naked with Phil. He touched me once, and I told him that I didn't like it and that he should stop. And he did stop, thank God.

But there were other boys who weren't so fortunate. Later, I heard accounts of how Mr. Bowen penetrated two of the boys after school in a back office. One of these victims would call me years later in a state of panic to tell me how much Mr. Bowen fucked up his life. There would be countless other victims before he was stopped.

For my part, I tried to set aside the man's weird side and ignore it while appreciating his kindness and skill as a teacher when we had our clothes on. I figured it would be too embarrassing to tell anyone about his weird side. It was something you just had to tolerate. My eight-year-old brain wasn't able to understand the damage he was doing, but a few of the other boys did the right thing and told their parents.

A few months into the fourth grade there was an abrupt change. My mother came into my room one night to tuck me in for sleep. But first she had something she needed to say. She told me that Mr. Bowen was fired "for playing with boys' private parts." Then she asked me if he ever played with mine.

"No," I said, "I don't know anything about it."

That night I cried hard in my mother's arms and couldn't sleep when she left the room. Then I put on a strong face to fight off the remaining tears. Enough is enough.

Next day at school I was greeted by a nondescript female teacher who stood there in place of Mr. Bowen. That was the day I stopped enjoying school. Maybe it was the same day I stopped trusting people in positions of authority.

My grade school probably wanted to save itself the embarrassment of public exposure. So without pressing criminal charges, they simply fired Mr. Bowen. They could have saved a lot of future victims, but they opted to save their reputation instead.

Meanwhile, he went on to teach at other schools where he continued to do the same treacherous things. After being fired from Christ Methodist, he took a job in Michigan where after several years he was fired again for molesting boys in his class. Then in the early 1980's, he and his wife chartered their own school in Ormond Beach, Florida. Of course, the same things happened and his wife apparently knew all about it. A restraining order was placed against Mr. Bowen, banning him from being on school property, but he violated the order just as he violated more and more boys. When he was finally arrested and the details of his career made public, Mr. Bowen would be considered the worst sex offender on record in the State of Florida.

In the late 1980's, after a drawn out legal battle, he was locked up for good in a Florida State Prison. In 1996, he was declared dead in a prison hospital after being sick with an un-disclosed illness. I suspect he was killed, although the article in the paper didn't specify. Known pedophiles don't last very long in prison.

Sitting alone in the day room I think about Mr. Bowen but I can't generate much anger toward the rotten bastard. Mostly I feel a sorrowful pity for the guy. It's a good start because it's the first time I've felt anything about him since the night my mother said he was fired. A fresh feeling of anger rises up and then passes just as quickly. I figure I need to stick with the agenda, which isn't Mr. Bowen but my father and his supposed neglect. Still, I feel an uneasiness creeping in again. Does my dad really deserve all the blame?

Maybe my father knows something isn't right when he

comes to visit me on the ward or when he takes me out for evening passes. The social workers have little to do with him when he's around, but they don't hold back when we're in therapy talking about him behind his back. No one invites my dad in to speak for himself. Maybe the staff knows how volatile such a meeting might be, or maybe they fear the repercussions of putting a prestigious doctor on the spot like that.

By this time I wonder why we haven't talked more about the incident that happened on my last day of high school and my feelings of guilt and shame over it. The staff knows about Lois and her 10-speed bicycle, but they don't question me about it beyond the facts of the case. It could be that it doesn't fit into their formulation of how I went crazy, so they don't factor it into their list of potential causes. But in fairness, I don't go out of my way to bring it up either. It's too shameful a thing to talk about.

13

A FEW days after the ordeal with the gay social worker, my sleep is back to normal and the nightmares gone. Well rested, I go down for recreational therapy with Arthur and some of the other patients.

Together, Arthur and I walk around the fitness track. He tells me about some of the hardships of his life and how he always managed to pull through. I ask him how he did it, and he says, "By doing just what we're doing now."

This sounds cryptic, so I ask him what he means.

"Walking, keep on walking," he says. "Whatever you do, that'll help."

I want to be polite, but this is the kind of simplistic nonsense I can do without. I complain about the drugs being forced on me, and I ask, "How could walking help with that?"

His response is that this is an even better reason to keep walking. "Walk off the drugs," he says.

I don't put much stock in Arthur's advice. It isn't profound for one thing—I want something deep and earthshaking. And who is he to profess wisdom in getting through hardship? Sure, he's an old man with a lot of experience over the years. But look at him—he's anxious as hell. He can barely hold a cup of coffee without spilling it all over his lap. His voice shakes when he speaks, and I never hear him say anything smart in group therapy. He's the kind of person you hardly ever notice.

Despite all this, his advice has a way of sticking with me. Maybe he has other pieces of wisdom to impart, but I'll never know. He's discharged the next day. He gets to walk the hell out of here.

By the 15th of March, three weeks after being admitted, I'm feeling more and more anxious to leave. The boredom is almost intolerable, especially when I compare my life to that of my friends at school. Phil, Deano and some of the fraternity brothers are coming down from Auburn for spring break. They're doing what I should be doing. It pisses me off to think that I have to stay here while they're living it up, soaking up sun and beer and getting it on with college girls. What the hell am I doing here anyway?

I talked with Dr. Frei a few days ago about getting discharged, and he agreed that if I remain stabilized I could go in a matter of days. Now, a few days later, it feels like I ought to be leaving today. To show what a good sport I am, I decide to wait until tomorrow at the latest.

As if to throw a wrench in my plans, Dr. Frei is away on vacation, and I don't know when he'll be back. Covering for him is another psychiatrist, Dr. Jordan, who seems more flexible. With him I talk more openly about my problems, including those with the medication. Because my blood pressure is getting dangerously low on the Thorazine, almost to the point of making me faint when I get up out of a chair, Dr. Jordan reduces the dose from 800 to 600 milligrams per day. This little move wins him points with me.

On the evening of the 15th I'm sitting in the day room, bored and wondering if the staff is just toying with me when they say I'll be leaving soon. I'm dead set on leaving tomorrow, and it's a testament to my self-control that I don't bolt from the place right now.

It's hard mustering the necessary patience. I've got to find something to ease my nerves. It occurs to me that I haven't read a book in over two months. There were a few *Readers' Digest* articles I've read here and there, which took all my concentration to finish. I want to challenge myself by reading a full-length book, but I don't want to set myself up for failure, so I search for the smallest book I can find.

I end up choosing *Jonathan Livingston Seagull*, by Richard Bach, which is really short and even has pictures. One of the younger patients says he's read the book 15 times and loved it just as much with each reading. I think he's a complete fool to read anything 15 times. "Get a life!" I want to tell him, but I don't say anything. Instead, I open the tiny volume and read in a quiet place.

I soon realize that it wouldn't be much of a stretch to read the thing 15 times. It's the perfect book for those with attention deficit disorder or for someone drugged up on neuroleptics. I finish the book by bedtime, feeling a good sense of accomplishment. After reading about this lone seagull, I start to think it's possible for people to fly, as long as they believe they can. Belief is the key. This feeds into another stream of thought, taking me to the image of Jesus walking on water. He could do it because he had perfect faith that he could. Then, after Jesus did it, his disciple Peter got cocky and figured he could replicate the feat. So Peter stepped out of the boat and took three steps on the surface—not a bad start—but then, *pfloom*, he plunged under the water. Jesus kind of scolded him when he said to Peter, "Oh ye of little faith."

So that's how it is, I think. Just have faith and everything will be okay. And as a bonus, maybe I could even fly or walk on water.

Next morning I get up and gather my belongings to go home. No one says today's the day, but I'm ready, and this is a free country. And it is the open ward after all.

Right after breakfast, I put my stuff in a Burdines shopping bag and make my way down the stairs. I half expect there to be sirens and bells sounding off, alerting a bunch of guards. But I'm able to leave the building undetected. Now I'm free to do whatever I want.

Walking down Federal Highway I think about Arthur and his advice. Maybe this is what he meant. Maybe he was trying to tell me I should walk my ass out of there. Only he was trying to be subtle about it to avoid getting into trouble.

I'm not sure where to go, but it doesn't take long to realize my options are limited. I have no money, and the flimsy bag I'm carrying won't hold up for a long walk. I think about going to the beach at Lauderdale-by-the-Sea to cool off in the surf. Maybe I could even test my faith by walking on water, but it's too long a walk from here. It doesn't occur to me to attempt flying.

With less lofty ideals in mind, I decide to do the natural thing under the circumstances. I go home.

As I approach the house, bag in hand, I realize that I don't have a key to get in, and since it's a weekday my mother and sister are sure to be gone. So I go around to the backyard patio and lie down on a lounge chair by the pool. Already the day is more excitement than any I've had in a while, and I don't have the energy to take it all in.

After a short nap I retrieve a pair of shorts from the shopping bag and change into them. Then, to clear away the remnants of sleep, I jump into the pool for a refreshing swim. I paddle around a couple of laps and get kind of bored. But soon my dip is interrupted.

First my mother emerges from the sliding glass door, then I hear sirens and see flashing blue lights of about three police cars parked in front of our house. The cops come jogging around the side yard to the patio, and they stand around the pool, poised for God-knows-what. It's a threatening sight from where I'm standing, and it could get worse if I put up a struggle. There're about five or six policemen here on my account. Jesus, you'd think they'd have something more worthwhile to do, like busting drug traffickers or something.

The cops try to look casual, like this is an everyday sort of thing for them. But to me it's a big deal. If I make one abrupt move, it could be target practice on my chest and a cloud of blood and flesh infusing the pool.

That's not what I had in mind for today. For one, my mother wouldn't be able to handle it. My going psycho is one thing—not an easy thing—but having my guts splayed all over the pool would be something else altogether. She doesn't deserve that.

So I stand motionless, letting my mother do the talking. Resisting the impulse to argue, I agree to let my mother drive me back to the hospital.

After a brief moment of drying off and changing clothes in my room, I'm back on the sixth floor of the Imperial Point Medical Center.

My rage is ready to materialize, but I know there's a seclusion room available for my occupancy and I doubt there's a shortage of cuffs and straps.

Just before bedtime my mother calls on the phone feeling guilty for bringing me back here, so she tries to apologize and explain why she did it. I don't want to hear her crap. The mere sound of her voice makes me madder by the second. I slam down the phone and tell the nurse I won't take any more calls tonight.

Next morning I get up and go through the tired monotony
of starting my day on the inpatient ward. It's hard, but the best
strategy is to be pleasant and agreeable. Don't ask about getting out. That'll only make it worse. They tack on extra days
for that kind of talk. I suppose when my insurance expires I'll
be free to go, but I have the good fortune of having one of
these *golden boy* policies with all sorts of extras.

As part of the morning ritual I visit with the psychiatrist,
Dr. Jordan in this case, since Frei is still on vacation. We talk
about yesterday's elopement from the hospital and about the
kind of thinking that led me to do it. I try my best to seem
normal and rational. Then Dr. Jordan says today was set as the
day for me to be discharged, but with this turn of events he
wonders whether it's a bad idea.

Now it's up to me to convince him otherwise. It's my shining opportunity—to demonstrate my sanity in such a way that
I can finally get out of here.

I'm not so sure I do a very good job in this regard. Dr. Jordan can probably see right through my candy-coated depiction
of how everything will be fine once I'm home. I tell him how
I'll get back on track by re-enrolling at Auburn and reconnect-
ing with old friends. I tell him I might even join the Auburn
Football team, which is ludicrous and pretty blatant as far as
grandiose delusions are concerned. We have the familiar talk
about medication, and I know better than to argue the point
about my needing to take it. I have to exercise monumental
self-control when Dr. Jordan uses the term *chemical imbalance* to describe my condition.

Whatever I said must have worked because Dr. Jordan
gives the green light for me to go. I'm sure he knows my judgment isn't the best, nor do my thoughts flow together in the
most rational way, but these are details that can be worked out
in a doctor's office. The main thing is that I'm not a threat for
going out and doing something stupid, like killing myself or

taking someone else's life.

I don't know it at the time, but my diagnosis at discharge and throughout my three week hospitalization is *acute schizophrenia*. No more pretending this is some adjustment reaction, like the way Dr. Jenkins put it. Now I have psychiatry's hallmark diagnosis. It's the same label affixed to the drooling vegetables and the glazed doughnuts, the ones who are perpetually in and out of state mental wards doped up on neuroleptics for life.

14

I T ' S Friday, March 17th, and I'm heading home. Besides taking the drugs and having regular outpatient sessions with Dr. Frei, there aren't any further plans. In the immediate future I want to join the Auburn group already here for spring break. Up to now it feels like life has been passing me by. Everyone but me is having a good time, leading productive lives. It's Phil I'm most envious of. He has life by the balls as far as I can tell. He's passing all his classes, dating pretty college girls, and he's made it through the fraternity's initiation. I don't even want to acknowledge what a great success he is because that would make me look even more pathetic. The best thing is to make up for lost ground and do it quickly. As such, being a part of the spring break group takes on a new sense of urgency.

Once home I make arrangements to get my car back. This is an essential first step, especially in Fort Lauderdale, which wasn't designed with the pedestrian in mind. The car is a barometer of freedom and status in this town, maybe more than anywhere else. My El Camino is like an old friend I haven't seen in a while, not since the day I packed my stuff at CDV. I didn't think about it much while at the hospital, but now it's like an obsession. A friend drove it down from Auburn for spring break, so I know it's around somewhere…but where?

After a little prodding, my mother lets it slip out that the car is parked at my father's house. She doesn't think I'm ready to drive it, citing medication as the main reason, but she's also worried about my judgment or lack thereof. We argue about it, but I'm not giving in. It's my car and I have a right to drive it.

Once her school day is over, I get Julia to take me over to dad's house so I can fulfill my mission. When we arrive, sure enough, the El Camino is parked out front on the street, looking as good as she ever did. My plan is to slip in and slip out as quickly as possible.

But I get sidetracked. My aunt, uncle and cousin are here visiting from Philadelphia. I can't be rude and ignore them, but I'm in no mood to sit down for a chat. There's also another thing playing heavily on my nerves—it's the fact that my aunt is a psychiatrist. I'm afraid she'll see right through me and maybe even recommend my going back to the hospital. This leads to frazzled nerves, which I know she can detect. But I've had some practice being pleasant and agreeable, despite what's below the surface.

As it turns out, I'm too agreeable for my own good. I agree to have dinner and spend the night at my dad's after returning from my night out with the guys. I also agree to let my 15-year-old cousin David tag along with me for the night.

Dinner is delicious, as always when my stepmother cooks. But by the time it's over I'm up to my eyeballs in pleasantries. It's like the scenario of the bull in the china shop, only I'm the china shop and they're all bulls. That's how it feels. But I could turn into the bull just as easily.

After dinner I call Phil to find out about tonight's plan. He says everyone is hanging out on his father's boat for the night, which sounds perfect to me. It's a familiar spot without too much commotion, a good place for me to get back on track. There's sure to be plenty of beer and maybe even some nice looking college girls. Life is starting to look good again.

With David as passenger, I drive back over to my house and park the car in the driveway. Then we make the short walk down to Phil's house.

The boat should be a fine place to be tonight. I've had some good times there and some bad times too, which I can laugh about now. First I should explain that it's not an ordinary motorboat. It's a 53-foot-long Hatteras cruiser with three staterooms at the bottom level, three bathrooms—or heads, they call them—a spacious galley midway up, and at deck level there's a plush salon with wall-to-wall carpeting, a couch and swivelling designer chairs. There's a fly bridge above the salon and a deck at the stern with a wet bar. A high quality sound system pipes music throughout the craft.

Phil's father is a wealthy man who made smart trades in the stock market in the 1960's. He was able to retire to South Florida at the age of 43 leaving behind a brokerage firm and a large office building in Manhattan bearing his initials. Despite the loss of his first wife, he's not exactly a guy you feel sorry for. He's now remarried to an attractive woman who shares his interest in yachting. Together they're living Florida's version of the American dream.

As a kid I joined Phil's family on boating trips, going to such places as the Bahamas and Key Largo. The trips started with Phil, his sisters and me all lying on the bow of the boat, sunning ourselves as we cruised to our destination. I never quite accepted the fact that I get sunburned by little more than a glancing shot of sun rays. A few hours into the trip Phil's stepmother would tell me that I looked like a lobster, which didn't do much to comfort me. The bad sunburn made the rest of the vacation a kind of stingy itchy hell. So alcohol was employed, and I don't mean topically.

At the age of 15, I didn't know how to handle the drink, and on one occasion I puked my guts out in my sleep. I slept on the top bunk in the bow stateroom with Phil's bunk below, set out slightly, matching the curve of the hull. I awoke with a bad hangover, only to see this mess of vomit down on the floor and on Phil's bed with him lying next to it. It looked like Phil was the guilty party from my vantage point, so I blamed him for it when he woke up. An argument followed.

But then, what puzzled me was this little portion of puke on my bunk. How do the laws of physics account for that? Obviously, they don't, and soon I was cleaning up the mess while trying to go undetected by Phil's father and stepmother. This happened on Easter Sunday, and Phil's stepmother had a nice little Easter egg hunt set up for us on the boat. How fortunate for me. There I was, hungover like a bitch, cleaning up puke, hiding the cleaning products, searching for Easter eggs and trying to look like a good sport. Life couldn't get much better.

My point in recounting all this is that I feel like I have proprietary rights to hang out on Phil's boat tonight. After all I've been through, and since I haven't seen these guys in two months, it feels right to have our reunion here.

David and I walk around the side yard to the dock behind Phil's house. We can hear music, talking and laughter coming from the boat. Phil and Deano are in the salon near the entry, surrounded by a bunch of fraternity brothers. A few college girls are here too, but I don't recognize any of them, which may be a good thing. It means they don't know about my recent history, and I'm not about to say anything. Hopefully no one else will blab about it either.

I'm shy when it comes to meeting women, rarely the one to make the first move and, fresh out of the mental ward, I don't have the confidence to change that pattern. It's best to stick with the familiar, so I talk with Phil and David.

It's clear that Phil has worries about me here on the boat. He knows I just got out of the hospital, and the last time he saw me I was kicking windows, punching Deano and preaching about how the Moon is God. Now I'm here on his boat drinking beer, acting like everything's fine. It's uncomfortable talking with him right now, so I step down to the galley hoping to make a better impression on the others. My first goal is to prove that my sanity is intact.

For a while things go well. I joke around and even make some people laugh. I say some nice things to one of the girls, who doesn't seem to mind, and I'm enjoying the buzz the beer is giving me. I think the night could turn out a success after all.

But then, in the midst of all this happy reunion feeling, I can hear one of the fraternity brothers in the salon talking about me. He's speaking to one of the girls while pointing over to me. He's telling her that I'm the psycho who nearly trashed the fraternity house.

My chest tightens at the sound of his pompous voice. And despite my fear, I walk closer to him, hoping my proximity will get him to shut the fuck up. But he isn't looking my way as he keeps yammering on. He tells the girl about how I was locked up in a nuthouse, which puts a look of disgust on her face. She looks around the room and her eyes settle on me with the same look of disgust.

I'm horrified but still hoping to avoid a scene. I call over to the pompous frat brother in a nerve-wracked voice. I say, "Greg, uh, would you come over here for a minute?"

"Yeah, in a couple of minutes," he says.

I stand and wait, feeling my anger multiply. I think of what I could do to this pencil-neck prick. I want to take his preppy face in my hands and pop it like a zit! I think about lunging at him with a barrage of fists to his face. But I fight off the impulse.

After what seems like an hour, Greg comes over to have a talk. He must have been thinking about what to say because it sounds like a prepared speech. He starts with the arrogant claim that I'm not welcome on the boat, like he's the new owner or something. He says the party is limited to "brothers only," and since I'm only a pledge I'm not included. Then he says that my cousin doesn't belong here either.

By this time we're attracting a crowd, but nobody is talking except for Greg, the pencil-neck prick. I think Phil realizes how close I am to plundering Greg's flesh, so he steps in to make peace. First he tries to reason with Greg and then with me, but neither of us is backing down. Then Phil leads me aside and tells me that it's probably best if David and I leave the party—no hard feelings. David agrees. Then Phil says something about Greg's being drunk as an excuse to justify his behavior. But none of this matters to me. The thing is, I now realize I'm standing alone with no one in my corner, not even my so-called best friend, and if I attack Greg now I'll really look like a psycho.

So without a word I walk off the boat.

As I gain some distance from the dock I start to feel pathetic, like I missed a golden opportunity to set things straight. It's partly about revenge over Greg, the pencil-neck prick, and yet it's more than that. It's all the rage that's been building over the past two months, and now even Phil has let me down. The molten lava starts to surface.

As David and I get to the front of the house, I see something I can't resist. It's Greg's new Mazda RX-7 shining under the street lamp, vanity plate and all.

It doesn't take much convincing before David and I engage in an act of vandalism. We twist the windshield wipers, kick the side of the car and knock off a side view mirror. When the damage seems sufficient, we run breathlessly back up the street to my house, jump in the El Camino and blast out of the neighborhood like a rocket. The gesture to Greg's car isn't as gratifying as I hoped, but it'll have to do for now.

By this time you might be wondering, and with good reason, whether I had a propensity for violent behavior before now. Truth is, I had only been in two fights my entire life, and I've never actually started a fight.

The first one happened when I was in the sixth grade at Fort Lauderdale Christian School. This eighth-grader named DW—no clue what it stood for—would come over and tease me to try to get me fired up. Even though he was two years older, he was also a couple of inches shorter than me, and he thought this was a terrible injustice that needed to be rectified. It's as if I was his superior by dint of height, and it was his duty to knock me down. But I didn't feel superior to him or anyone else back then, so I didn't understand his gripe with me.

One day after school DW challenged me to a fight behind the new gymnasium, having spread word of the fight beforehand. When I arrived, a group of students (mostly eighth-graders) had already formed a circle.

Petrified with fear I stood back, far behind the circle and away from DW. I had no idea what to do, but I knew I didn't want to earn the label of being a chicken. DW signaled me to come into the circle with him, and he might have said a thing or two about the fight, but I was too scared to comprehend.

Seconds later he started dancing around, punching me all over and kicking me in the nuts. I tried to get into a decent stance and then I went after him with a couple of punches to the chest. DW wore glasses, and I thought it would be too cruel to damage them, so I avoided hitting him in the face. But DW had no restrictions on where to hit me. In a few minutes I had blood streaming out of my nose, which prompted one of the kids in the circle to call the fight over.

On the drive back home from school, my mother looked all worried and asked me what happened. All I could say was, "I should've hit him in the face!"

Back home in my bedroom, I closed the door and put a small pillow on a chair, pretending it was DW's face, glasses and all. I punched and punched and punched the pillow, all the while yelling, "Hit him in the face! Hit him in the face! Hit him in the face!" No way would I allow myself to forget the lesson.

Flash forward three years to the ninth grade—freshman year at Cardinal Gibbons—to a nearly identical situation. This time it was a 10th-grader named Tom Noel who again was shorter than I, as almost everyone was. Tom prided himself as a tough guy, and he thought of me as a big klutzy freshman who could barely find the seat of his pants, which wasn't far from the truth. Every day in school, when we passed each other between classes, he'd call me names like *doofus* or *nerd* or the worst, *lurch*. The guy seemed like a wild animal to me, not someone to mess with. I took the insults without looking at him and without breaking my stride. But he didn't like being ignored, so he increased his threats. I knew a fight was coming.

One day, nervous as hell, I walked out of Spanish class, taking the familiar route to seventh period Religion. I knew Tom was planning to jump me, and this would be when he'd do it. I walked like a block of wood along the outdoor corridor and as predicted Tom attacked, jumping on my back and twisting me to the ground. On my knees, I was hit by a flurry of punches while trying to get up. Slowly, I worked my way up, but I kept slipping because of the goddamn slick boots I was wearing. By the time I finally assumed my feet, there was a crowd forming a circle around us, just like in the sixth grade. This is pack animal behavior, and I guess it's a human trait too. Tom had his set of cheerleaders and I had mine.

Soon the memory of DW returned and, with it, the lesson. I started following Tom's head as it bobbed and weaved around on his neck. My focus sharpened as I moved in. I landed a few hard shots to his face and head while protecting mine. After a series of good pops, Tom lowered his head and tried to cover himself, backing away into the crowd.

But I wasn't done. This was for DW too. I went after any portion of exposed head I could find, knocking him side-to-side, feeling the support of my cheering section.

Then Dean Green came in and broke the thing up. He yelled at me and Tom and told everyone else to go back to class. Dean Green was a big beefy sort of guy you didn't want to mess with, in addition to the fact that he was the dean after all. He grabbed Tom and me by the armpits and thrust us forward, directing us to his office whereupon he demanded handshakes and apologies on both sides.

Tom gave me no trouble after that, and I felt a debt of gratitude to DW. It's true what they say about learning things the hard way. You don't forget those lessons.

The next year I took a few boxing lessons, figuring there might be more DWs or Tom Noels in the world. I also put up a heavy bag and a speed bag in the garage for practice. But until the madness of this year, I've never considered attacking someone without first being provoked.

Back at my father's house, I spend a fitful night sleeping on a rollaway bed. After breakfast I drive back to my house, figuring I should spend a little time with my mother. There's always this feeling of guilt whenever I think I'm spending more time with my dad than with my mother. I have to keep their time allotment in proper balance to be a good son and all. Neither parent puts a guilt trip on me, not consciously at least, but I can sense the tension. The feelings of hurt are stronger on my mother's side, since she was the one scorned, so I feel as though she needs a stronger alliance from me. When I'm with her I make a point of not saying anything complimentary about dad. If she says something cutting about him, I stay quiet, or if I'm upset with him too I give a nod of agreement. To a lesser degree, the same thing happens at my father's house with the roles reversed.

I drive back to my house late in the morning still angry as hell over what happened last night. Despite the vandalism, none of the anger has left me. In fact it's intensified. I still want to beat the crap out of Greg, and I still feel betrayed by Phil and the others on the boat. To them I'm like a freak show. The women on board must have felt relieved when I left—no more worries about being paired up with a psycho.

My intention, as always, is to keep these thoughts and feelings to myself. Let others know they've got the upper hand and they'll whack you with it. And don't let anyone see you lose control. Wait long enough and maybe the tables will turn. But the problem is that I don't have the patience or self-control to hold back the flood of emotion. It's not a good situation. The lava is ready to flow.

Sometimes it's just a word or the way a thing is said that sets things in motion. It's a mysterious thing really. Emotions form into action. I don't know what my mother says to trigger it. Maybe she doesn't say anything but only looks at me with that concerned, motherly look, the kind that speaks for itself. It says, "I'm here if you want to talk." It says, "I care about you, and I'm concerned." It also tells me that it's safe to let her know what's going on. "No one will hurt you here," it says. But her look gives no warning of the dangerous shit bubbling up inside me. That's a message I don't get.

So in the comfort of my home, with my mother standing by, I proceed to let the lava erupt. First I yell full-throated until my voice is shot. Then I commence smashing things in my room. I tell my mother how much I hate everything and everyone and how I wish the whole fucking lot of them would go to hell! I grab the *étagère*, which is a fancy way of saying goddamn bookcase, and swing it down hard on the floor with the contents springing to life. Then I smash everything in the bookcase that isn't already broken. I keep smashing things, and I want to smash more things. The world doesn't have enough things in it for me to smash. That's the problem.

On it goes for the better part of the afternoon. Among the more costly item destroyed is the stained glass window encased in the front door. I put my fist through it as if it were a piece of aluminum foil.

My mother, who can be pretty fearless when she wants to be, watches me do all this without reacting too much. She knows better than to call the cops or insist on another admission to the hospital just now. Instead, she takes it upon herself to calm me in her motherly way.

I'm up the entire night, and my mother stays up with me. By 3 A.M. I'm worn out but still mad, like a rabid animal. I say to my mother, "I could easily break everything in this house."

"I know you can," she responds, "but you won't, right?"

I take the wiser route and keep my bloody hands idle for now. I think maybe I should sleep, but I'm wound up too tight, and my bed is littered with broken glass anyway. I'm in no mood to clean it up. Instead of sleeping, I sit in the family room, staring wild-eyed at nothing in particular.

By dawn I fix upon a plan of action. I realize there's no place for me here in Fort Lauderdale—no decent job, no girlfriend and no college worth attending. Phil doesn't seem to want me around, and I'm probably the laughing stock of the fraternity. All my other high school friends are either working or are far away at school. And I'm still mad at my father but not willing to talk about it. My mother, despite all her support, has the propensity for delivering me to the nuthouse. So even though it's still spring break, my plan is to drive up to Auburn and get my life straightened out up there.

I still have the image of the all-night diner where I meet with the gallery of prophets. It's there that I'm supposed to get messages from the other world. This is surely not happening in South Florida.

In preparation for the trip I pack a few things, including my Walkman, but fail to include many of the items necessary for a 650-mile journey and who-knows-what beyond that. I pack one or two changes of clothing, no toiletries and no money.

Also notably absent is the Thorazine everyone tells me I need in order to maintain mental stability. All it does is dull me out and lower my blood pressure. So I walk over to the side yard of our house and toss the contents of the bottle over the fence, onto our next door neighbor's lawn. I hope their dog Topper doesn't get too curious milling around in the grass. He deserves better than to ingest that crap.

I don't tell my mother about my plan to drive to Auburn, figuring she'll do something stupid like toss my keys in the canal or something, but she can tell I'm up to no good. She saw me packing, and she saw me toss the medication. As a kind of last ditch effort to spoil my plans before calling the cops, she gives her friend Ron a ring and frantically tells him to come over. He arrives shortly thereafter, but his presence at the house is little more than a mild nuisance. When I'm ready to go, keys in hand, I walk through Ron, shoving him to the side when he tries to stop me. I kick open the windowless front door, sprinting to the El Camino.

Traveling west on Commercial Boulevard and then north on the Florida Turnpike, I'm happy again. It's the joy that comes from making my own decisions without obstacle. The fact that I have no money and only a third of a tank of gas doesn't impede my mood. I'm free, and that's what matters. I blast the stereo and push the accelerator down near the floor.

My brain is buzzing as the car cruises at over 90 miles an hour. We're in harmony.

The image of Jonathan Livingston Seagull resurfaces, and I think of my El Camino as the lone seagull. If she runs out of gas—no problem—the car will take to the open skies. Let's see the cops pull me over then.

It's the magical world again, but it seems completely logical to me. In the magical world things have a soul, just like a person does, and inanimate objects can communicate with other objects and even with people, but only with people who have the inner knowing. For sure I have the inner knowing, like Luke Skywalker and the Jedi Knights. I could divine my El Camino into flight with an empty gas tank, easy. And what's the point of money? The magical world doesn't respond to something as petty as the forces of capitalism. People who still use money as a means of exchange are weak-minded, easy prey for the likes of me. I'll apply some mental force to the situation and people will gladly give me what I require. That's how it works. Soon I'll have an opportunity to test these new ideas.

Near the exit for the coastal town of Stuart my car starts coughing, and after about a half-mile the engine sputters to a stop. I let the car coast on the shoulder of the highway for the length of a football field and stop when I'm next to one of the blue emergency call boxes. What a terrific piece of good fortune, I think, and I thank God for the gift. I get out, walk over to the call box and pull down the white lever. I half expect to hear the voice of the Almighty transmitting instructions on how to save my soul and that of the El Camino. But instead there's a weak voice asking me what the problem is.

"I ran out of gas. Can you help?" I ask.

The voice sounds irritated when it responds, "We'll send someone over."

Okay, fine, not exactly infinite wisdom but at least it's

something.

Ten minutes later, a redneck looking guy with a baseball cap and teeth missing pulls up in a Sunoco tow truck. He lifts out a dirty red tank and walks over to my car without saying anything. I'm sitting on the open tailgate with the gas cap next to me. I show him to the nozzle into which he pours the contents of the tank, probably no more than a gallon.

I read deeper meanings into the situation, like this gasoline exchange is some kind of new communion among spiritual brothers—blood of Christ and stuff like that. The redneck doesn't seem to share my affinity for things spiritual. He wants money, cash money, and he wants it now. But I figure what he really wants, and what he needs, is a firm handshake from a fellow soul traveler. So that's what I give him. Then I get back in my car and drive on.

By this time I'm not as confident of my old El Camino taking flight, and I figure she'll probably require more gasoline for the balance of the trip. Up ahead I see a sign for the Fort Pierce Service Plaza and decide it's a good idea to fill up there.

Funny thing is, the redneck guy in the Sunoco truck followed me here, and he doesn't have the look of satisfaction on his face I expected my handshake would give him. In fact, he looks pretty pissed off. He's at the next fill-up island talking with the manager of the station, looking over at me while he's talking. Meanwhile I fill my tank as fast as I can. The disturbing fact starts settling in that I have no money and no credit card, and these are important items here on the turnpike. It seems a handshake won't suffice. I decide not to wait around for the inevitable. I jump back in the car, tank half-filled, and ride off.

With this new set of experiences fresh in mind, my confidence is shaken. The thing to do now is haul ass up to Auburn where I still believe I'll find my little slice of heaven. And haul ass is what I do. When I pass the state trooper parked in the median strip, my clocked speed is 95 miles an hour, which is 40 over the posted speed limit. I hit the brakes but the damage is done. The familiar flashing blue lights strobe in my rear view mirror. "Goddammit!" I yell out loud. Then, like a good citizen, I pull over onto the shoulder.

The trooper tells me to stay in the car, but by the time he says it I'm already halfway out and I don't have the nerve to sit back down and wait. It's clear that he doesn't like this. "Sit your ass back down in the car," he says, "and put your hands on the wheel."

Then another trooper pulls up. I'm curious why all the fuss, and I guess I don't get back in the car as fast as I should because the cop changes his order. He tells me to face the side of the car and lean forward with my hands and legs spread apart. I do as instructed and ask why he's making this into such a big deal.

He tells me to shut up and says he'll ask the questions from now on.

I don't move from the required position while the troopers search my El Camino. One of the cops asks why I stole the gas, and why was I going so fast? Where the hell was I going anyway? I have no suitable answers, as far as they're concerned. By the time we get to the third question—the one about where I was going—I figure I'm a goner. I have the sense not to mention the gallery of prophets, but the first thing that comes to mind isn't much better. I say I was headed to a mental hospital in Alabama.

As soon as the words come out, I know it's a bad move. Now I'm screwed for sure. One of the troopers frisks me while the other watches like a hawk. I start getting angry, telling the cop not to frisk me so hard.

"Boy, I'll frisk you any way I want," he says.

I can feel my face turning red with rage. I probably don't

need to state the obvious, but of all places to be enraged this is not the recommended place. This isn't my home with mom looking on as I smash things. This is Florida Redneck Country with two cops and no witnesses. I should have the sense to shut up, but I don't. One of the cops takes my head and forces it down so my face presses sideways on the hot hood of the El Camino. My knees almost buckle from the pain. With my face burning, the other trooper handcuffs my wrists behind my back. I start to cry. Then both cops walk me over to the back seat of one of the trooper cars. I feel hands pushing me into the car. Then the door is shut. In a matter of seconds, they've reduced me to a sobbing, slobbering mess.

I sit in the blazing heat for half an hour while they discuss the situation with the highway patrol headquarters. There's a lot of talk going back and forth, which I can't make sense of from here. Soon another police car shows up, and then I see a flatbed tow truck backing up toward my El Camino. "What a mess!" I say to myself, "What a fucking mess."

Two cops get in the front seat of the car and we drive across the highway over the grassy median to the southbound side. I look back and see my car being pulled up with a cable onto the flatbed. It's one of the saddest sights I can imagine.

As we drive past the familiar service plaza, the cop in the passenger seat is making finishing touches on the police report. Then he tries to hand me a copy of the summons, which I can't reach. "I'm handcuffed," I say, "how am I supposed to get that?"

He smiles a little bit, realizing that I have a point. His next statement isn't what I had hoped to hear. He says, "I'll give it to you when we get to the hospital."

Jesus, here we go again.

15

OUR first destination is the emergency room of the Lawnwood Medical Center in Fort Pierce, where a nurse takes a blood sample, and another person conducts a mental status exam. Then, after I'm deemed certifiable, it's off to the Indian River Mental Health Center.

The facility is a single floor, cinder block and stucco structure near the main highway. It's in a rough section of town, whatever town this is, and it's clear that there'll be no gallery of prophets here. The place is small, and there aren't many people around because it's Sunday, which means they're short on staff. After the routine check-in, including a no-nonsense physical and the standard speech about rules and the schedule, a nurse ushers me to a stark room and points to my bed.

Unbeknownst to me, the head nurse has contacted my mother, who was able to get Dr. Frei's authorization to crank up the drugs again. Meanwhile, Dr. Frei and my parents are putting together a court petition to have me committed against my will, or *Baker Acted*, as per Florida State law. So in the span of no more than two hours, I've gone from the heights of freedom to the pit of gloom, hit hard by the double-barreled machine of the legal system and psychiatry.

Pow! Pow!

In a daze I walk around the facility trying to get my bearings. The day room is a combined dining area and recreation room, which has a door leading out to an open field. There's an orderly sitting by, monitoring the door for potential escapees. To run now would be foolish, and where would I go anyway? I don't even know where the hell I am. I wasn't paying attention when the cops brought me here. This could be Vero Beach, Stuart or any of a number of towns along the Gold Coast.

Not bent on leaving, I take a seat away from others in the day room where I watch patients. A middle-aged man has visitors with him, probably family, who've brought him a snack he doesn't seem to want. Maybe if I look his way long enough they'll offer me the food. The only thing I've had today was a lousy bowl of Cheerios.

Then I notice one of the strangest looking guys I've ever seen. He's a tall hulking man with flaming red hair shooting out like an Afro—only he's pasty white. He has a flat face with his forehead protruding out beyond his nose. And he's got this hideous scar just above his eyes, which looks like the product of a botched brain surgery.

I've heard about the frontal lobotomy in my psychology class, and I think this guy must've had it done to him. He walks in slow motion, stiff as mahogany, and his speech is a monotone, garbled mess. I can make out a couple of words here and there, and I fake like I understand the rest so as not to piss him off. To me he's the embodiment of Frankenstein.

A curious thing is that this guy is playing pool, or at least he's humoring himself by poking the stick at the pool balls in random fashion. He isn't causing any trouble at the pool table, but it occurs to me that, if he wanted to, he could cause some major damage. He's got plenty of ammunition with the sticks and pool balls. Jesus, if I say something to provoke him, I might get a striped or a solid cracked across my forehead, and then I'd be just like him, minus the Afro. Thankfully, the guy's disposition is mellow and he seems to have pretty good judgment. On the other hand, I wonder about the judgment of the staff for having a goddamn pool table here in the first place.

Frankenstein sees me sitting alone and looking bored, so he grunts for me to join him in a game of pool. I'm a lousy pool player, which is probably a good thing because I won't come off as a threat. We shoot around the table for a little while and then rack up for real game. It's an old table where the balls get stuck along the tracks at various places. I walk around and gather the balls, but Frankenstein gives me a sign to stop, like I'm wasting my effort. Then he stands at one end and squats, lifting the table up about a foot off the ground. You can hear the balls rolling down the rails until they come clacking to a halt. He shakes the thing for good measure to loosen any stubborn ones.

The technique impresses me, so after we shoot around again I try it myself. With tremendous strain, I commence raising the table but can only lift it several inches before having to set it back down, lest I pull a groin or something. Frankenstein looks proud when I defer the task back to him. We could've used this guy at the furniture moving company, although he might've scared off the customers.

After supper I get phone calls from my mother and father, both checking to see if I'm okay. Most of what we talk about is the standard perfunctory crap. Both my parents are concerned that they'll set me off, so they keep the conversation light and upbeat. My dad is uncomfortable chatting for more than a few minutes, so he hands the phone over to my aunt, the psychiatrist. She talks to me in a sweet tone, like I'm a kid, which rubs me the wrong way. I can feel the nerves rising. But before it gets out of hand, she turns the phone over to my cousin David, which means I have to go through yet another round of bullshit pleasantries.

This phone passing ritual is a family tradition, assuring that everyone stays in the loop. I don't mind it for holidays and reunions, but it's not a welcome thing now. By the time David gets on the phone I have no idea what to talk about, and I don't think he does either. What are you supposed to say to someone who's just gone nuts and landed himself in the wacko ward? Almost anything you say takes you down a bad road.

After the phone call I amble back to the day room.

The next day is Monday, March 20th, with full staff on hand. I take the day's first dose of Thorazine without protest, but things degenerate from there.

By mid-morning, I consider the ramifications of being locked up in this place with no car, no Walkman and no knowledge of where the hell I am or how long I have to stay. And just as before, they're authorized to pump me up with the same mind-numbing drugs. Should I sit back and take it like a nicey-nice patient? This is what everyone wants me to do. But do they really have my best interests at heart? Of course they say they do, but prison guards might well say the same thing. Actually, being in prison would be better than this. At least there they don't deliberately fuck with your biochemistry.

During lunch, a nurse presents me with my second daily dose of Thorazine. She's a short, fat troll of a woman with a dotted face. I tell her I'd rather not take the drug, pulling back from the table as I say this. I walk away, leaving most of my food behind. But the nurse follows me.

The floor plan of the building allows me to walk around in an oval, from the day room past the offices and bedrooms to the front waiting area and back around to the day room again through a different corridor. So I commence walking round and round in a counterclockwise fashion with the fat nurse following and then giving up after one round. The vigorous walking rouses me into a state of righteous anger.

During one of my passes through the waiting room, I knock off the plastic housing over the thermostat, and I kick it like a hockey puck.

Newly alerted, three of the male attendants chase after me, forcing me to reverse direction. One gets hold of my arm, but I twist it away without looking at him and then resume walking. It feels good to walk with this kind of intensity. The staff maintains pursuit, trying to get me to go voluntarily into the seclusion room. I refuse, and for a while I think I have my way.

Then three police officers come in through the front door and lock it behind them. I hadn't planned for this, and it forces me to change strategy. I sprint toward the far end of the day room, near the pool table. I consider the pool-table-equipment-as-weaponry option, but there aren't any balls or sticks here now.

The cops and a couple of male orderlies surround me. I get it in my head that they're going to kill me as soon as they catch me, which puts me in a state of desperate fear. With no other alternative, I dart through an opening toward the waiting area, but now they've closed off both corridors. One cop blocks me long enough for the others to catch up. Then they all grab parts of me while I'm flailing around like a maniac. At one point, my left arm gets free long enough to pop an attendant on the side of his head. This forces the rest of them to tighten their grip.

The short fat nurse returns with a syringe. I try staring her down with the most evil look I can muster.

"Don't you look at me that way!" she says.

So I stare at her harder, in a more sinister way. Maybe it'll be like *The Wizard of Oz* where the wicked witch melts away if the stare is strong enough. But no such luck. The nurse follows the men as they drag me into the seclusion room, and she watches as they strap me down to the bed in four-point restraints. Now I'm hers for the taking. One of the cops covers my face with a towel to break the evil eye contact. Meanwhile, two of the attendants twist my body and pull my shorts down to expose enough ass for the shot. As the nurse plunges in the contents of the syringe, I let out a shriek and proceed to call her every filthy name I can think of.

Sleep follows soon after the injection. Then I lie for hours in a stupor, mostly looking out the window. The fact that there's a window makes it odd for a seclusion room, or maybe it's a regular room designated for this purpose on special occasions. It doesn't matter. What matters is that I'll be spending the rest of the day and night here, cooped up like an animal.

There are dark clouds rolling in, and I can hear the trees whipping and whistling in the wind. A lone dog barks through the distance, maybe warning about the approaching storm. Soon cracks of thunder and lightning dominate the sky, followed by a downpour the likes of which I haven't seen in months, maybe years. My window vantage is the perfect place to take it in without getting wet. I'm a captive audience.

Normally storms in South Florida come and go in minutes, but this one lingers, and I'm grateful for it. It breaks up the boredom and takes me back to a better time, reminding me of summers I worked as a mason's tender in 1979 and '80. I got the job at the age of 14 from a mason who was hired to build a wall around my father's house. It seemed like a good way to earn money and stay in shape over the summer, better than vegetating in front of the tube.

The workday started early at a convenience store, where the masons bought cigarettes and coffee, and the laborers bought fresh pairs of work gloves to handle the concrete blocks. Everyday we bought a new pair of gloves and by the end of the day they were tattered rags.

The routine of the day was to stack blocks, right side up, in uniform piles across the length of the future wall. At roughly 10-foot intervals you put a wet board on top of a waist-high stack of blocks, and there you shoveled out the mortar, or mud, as they called it. Off to the side of the slab, you made the mud by mixing a combination of sand, water and Portland cement. If you screwed up the mixture, you might as well walk off the construction site because you wouldn't hear the end of it from the masons. Even if you made a good batch, some of the masons still complained. If there wasn't enough water, they called it *hard shit*, and if there wasn't enough sand, they called it *soupy shit*. So then you had to go over to the mason with a wheelbarrow and remix the mud with a shovel, adding the right amount of water or sand. If you spent too much time mixing, someone was sure to yell at you, and there was likely a mason running low on block. An idle mason meant you weren't doing your job. So you shoveled out the mud as fast as you could, then you ran over to the loudmouth mason to give him his block. And if you didn't stack them right-side-up, you might get a wet trowel mark across your ass.

When the wall got high enough, matters were further complicated by the use of scaffolding. Here you connected rails to the pins in a crisscross fashion and stacked the squared scaffolding units up as high as they needed to go. Next you set planks across the scaffolding for the entire length of the wall. Once set up, you tossed the blocks up there, going plank-to-plank, and then you shoveled up the mud to the wet mortarboards. If by this time your hands were bloody and blistered from the blocks, and your muscles ached or whatever, you knew not to complain about it to the masons. Their ridicule was enough to send you packing for the Everglades to live out your days with the alligators. They called you *pretty boy* and said they'd set you up with a manicure or a masseuse and stuff like that. Then they'd laugh like crazy and tell you to bring up the fucking mud.

There were days at the construction site when the skies turned an ominous gray. Thunder and lightning and hard thrusts of rain would blow in and send the masons running for cover. Throughout summer, you could almost count on it happening daily by late afternoon, and what a blessing it was for us laborers. I was paid by the hour, so this was time on the clock, time to sit back and do nothing but watch the rain and recuperate. Sometimes I joked with the masons, and once in a while one of them would give me a cold beer out of his cooler, which was nice.

Lying here, staked down to the bed in seclusion, my senses are soothed by the storm, and my thoughts drift back and forth between my current predicament and the construction memories. The dog isn't barking anymore. Now it's only the skies crackling with noise. The wild intensity of it shows me that there are some things stronger than the big egos controlling this God-forsaken place. If a storm can stop a bunch of headstrong masons, then maybe it can help me get out of here. I don't know how that could happen—logic isn't a part of my equation—but I believe God is behind the storm, and it's His way of sending me a loving message. If so, I'm listening.

16

T HE plan is to have me transferred to another hospital in Fort Lauderdale where Baker Acted patients are accepted. I know it won't be Imperial Point because it's not authorized for such patients, but I don't know where. It has to be a place where Dr. Frei has admitting authority.

The head nurse arranges for an ambulance to transport me. Just prior to my departure, she gives me another shot of Thorazine—one for the road, I guess.

The place they take me to is a plain looking structure on East Las Olas Boulevard, not far from the beach or the downtown business center. The nearest feature is the ritzy Las Olas shopping district, about a block up the street, where you see gaudy rich people and artsy types walking around with shopping bags. This is prime South Florida real estate. You couldn't find a more desirable business location, yet what a waste this place would prove to be.

The building bears the nondescript name *Fort Lauderdale Hospital*, and from the looks of it you wouldn't know what it is. It's a five story concrete structure painted beige with brown accents and flying buttresses on the north side of the building. The fifth floor was added soon after the place was built in the early 70's, which may explain the buttresses, though I'm not sure how. Whatever the case, it looks like a shoddy piece of architecture. Like it or not this is my home for the foreseeable future.

After the ambulance drops me off, I'm shown to an office on the first floor where a woman interviews me. I don't remember the encounter except for one short exchange. The woman asks how it is that I ended up here at the hospital. I tell her about the episode on Phil's boat and the violent aftermath. I can tell she's only half listening, and when I'm finished she says, "Well that's a hell of a way to spend spring break!" The way she says it is belittling and smart-ass, and it hits a raw nerve. I want to tell her off, but I'm all locked up inside and don't say anything.

After the standard preliminary stuff, including yet another physical, they assign me a room on the fifth floor. It's the adult locked ward where they put the more hard-core patients and the ones like me who are likely to escape. Downstairs on the second floor is the open unit for higher functioning adults who can leave the building with permission. In between, on the third and fourth floors, are the units for the addicts and the adolescents.

During the first day or so of my incarceration on the fifth floor, I give little evidence of a fuss. When medication is doled out at the standard times, I wait by the nurses' window and take it as directed. I attend group therapy and most of the activities offered by the staff. Other than these diversions I keep to myself, away from other patients, all of whom appear severely disturbed. The most desirable thing is to sleep, so I nap after meals and after medication. The sleeping is the best part of the day.

After a couple of days, I'm granted family visits. My mother shows up almost everyday, and my dad and sisters also come on a regular basis. On the third day, I get transferred downstairs to the open ward on the second floor. Apparently, I'm making steady progress—*good behavioral control, pleasant to be with and compliant with unit rules.* These are the observations recorded by staff. The fact that I'm emotionally flat, depressed, oversleeping and vegetating most of the day away doesn't appear to be a problem. To the staff and Dr. Frei, I'm on the road to stability.

A minor glitch in this steady progress is the fact that my blood pressure is dangerously low again with the Thorazine. I nearly faint whenever I get up, and I'm always lightheaded. So Dr. Frei lowers the dose while starting a different, more potent drug called Prolixin.

On the seventh day I go on my first outing with a group of patients and three social workers. The staff figures I'm not at risk for running away.

Up the street is a special event. It's the Las Olas Art Festival where the street is cordoned off for pedestrians only. The boulevard is taken over by a series of booths with arts and crafts from local vendors. It's a colorful sight, filled with attractive people. The stuff for sale is mostly of the tacky variety, possibly rejects from the Swap Shop flea market. I follow the group, looking back and forth between the stuff on display and the women, mostly looking at the women.

Nothing makes much of an impact on me until I recognize a couple of familiar faces. It's two of the female social workers from Imperial Point, and it looks like they've spotted me. "Oh shit!" I say to myself as they approach.

They both smile at me, and one of them asks, "Who are you here with?"

I don't know what to say. Do I tell them I'm back in another psycho ward, out for a walk, and then incur the look of pity on their faces? No, I can't take that right now. There's shame in just thinking about it. Instead I say, "I'm here with a couple of friends. We're kind of in a rush."

They can probably see right through me, but they don't say anything. And I'm grateful to avoid the look of pity. I cut the conversation short and charge ahead to be with the group. It's the safest thing.

Now that I've been in the hospital awhile, I know what to expect and I learn to play by the rules. The routine is a dull cycle of eat, sleep, take drugs and attend therapy sessions. Sometimes I listen to my Walkman or play Ping-Pong with another patient when there's nothing else going on, but the pull of sleep is always strong. Passes and visits with my family follow a regular rhythm as well, but there's a dwindling supply of things for us to talk about. Outside of sleeping, my most enjoyable form of relief is the milkshake my mother brings me two or three times a week. It's a tasty treat, but after it's gone it only adds to my sense of being a lazy, fat cat with no aim in life.

By the 1st of April, I start asking about getting discharged from the hospital. From the way it looks, everything is going well, right on schedule. Of course Dr. Frei is the one I have to convince, but even he seems to be softening to the idea. At first he says, "I'll look into it," which is about as close as I get to a full fledged commitment. In our next session he tells me I need a "longer period of stability." How long exactly, he won't say, and what constitutes stability, he won't say either. Dr. Frei is a master of the vague and the oblique. His wishy-washy language frustrates me, and I wonder what I have to do to get a firm answer.

On the morning of April 3rd, I can't take it anymore. There was talk about my getting out today, but Dr. Frei set the date forward another week. I think they're toying with me, just as they did at Imperial Point. But I won't stick around to play their games.

In my room I take the unused plastic bag out of the trash can and stuff my things into it. Slinking down low, with my bag draped across my back like Santa Claus, I pass the nurse's station and make my way to the west stairwell. To my maximum relief, the door leading outside is unlocked.

Heading west on Las Olas, I find a pay phone in front of a convenience store and dial the number of a high school friend named Bill. He's the only person I know who isn't away at school or working. You could say that Bill isn't the most ambitious sort. He's smarter than most, but his life is mostly about pulling pranks, drinking beer, smoking pot, and if asked he could do the best Jim Morrison imitation around. I can hear him now, stoned to the point of euphoria, with his hand cupped like a microphone singing:

Don't ya love her madly
Wanna be her daddy
Don't ya love her face
Don't ya love her as she's walkin' out the door
Like she did one thousand times before

Ten or so minutes after the call, a smiling Bill rolls up in a borrowed car. "Hey man, what's up?" he says.

Without pause I get in the car and we're off to his apartment. When we arrive, I see his brother sitting on a bean bag chair with a full leg cast and crutches alongside him. The place is on the second floor with no elevator, so I wonder how the brother gets up and down. I feel kind of sorry for him. He's sitting in the corner drinking a can of Budweiser, watching TV and he seems content. I ask him what happened with the leg, and he tells me the story, but I'm not really listening. Then he hands me a can of beer without asking whether I want it. At first I think it's a bad idea to drink with the medication and all that crap, but then I get into the good feeling of the moment.

I drink the beer and then another, and by the end of the second beer I'm feeling a good buzz. It's only the second time I've had alcohol since the episode at the Hungry Hunter with Deano and the Indian. Now I don't want to talk about the Moon or God or anything like that. But there's another kind of magical spell happening. By the middle of the third beer, I'm convinced I have the power to heal the broken leg. The only problem would be cutting off the cast. The thing is, I don't tell anyone about this magical power, and I don't do any laying-on of hands or anything like that. Instead, I let the thought pass without saying anything. Best to keep a low profile for now.

I get to thinking about where I'll sleep in this cubbyhole of an apartment. There are three of us, and the only place for me is a tiny love seat. While Bill and his brother are talking, I'm thinking of ways to contort my body to find a comfortable position on the couch. I figure if I'm tired enough I can sleep anywhere.

Then the phone rings, and Bill picks up. I give him a signal to make sure he knows I'm not here if anyone asks. Dutifully, Bill says, "He's not here" to the voice on the other end, which is the panic-stricken voice of my mother.

She tells him about my escape and how worried she is and how he must contact her right away if he hears anything. My mother goes on and on, repeating herself the way nervous mothers do. The call is only a few minutes, but it feels like an hour. Bill looks spent when it's done.

After he hangs up, I'm wracked by the same tension my mother just piled on Bill. We talk about what a creep he feels like for lying to my mother and about what I'm supposed to do now that she's all freaked out. The conversation shifts between my mother's panic, Bill's guilty feeling and my plan to avoid further incarceration. I'm straining my brain to come up with a plan to satisfy all sides.

About 20 minutes later the phone rings again, and Bill picks up again. No surprise—it's my mother. Bill's voice has more tension in it than I've ever heard, which makes me think of my mother's voice, and soon I can't take it anymore. I figure it'll never end. She'll call day and night, worried to hell, begging for morsels of information. Every time the phone rings it'll be instant anxiety and more lies.

I grab the phone and produce a monotone "Hello mom." Then I tell her my one demand, which is that I'll come home, but there's no way I'll agree to go back to that shit-hole of a hospital, nor any other such place. My mother checks with a couple of other people I can hear in the background—it sounds like a convention over there—and then tells me I can come home. To be sure, I have to verify that she means *for good*.

"Yes, that's right," she says.

I grab the trash bag with my stuff and head home in Bill's borrowed car. When we arrive, I invite Bill to come in. But he declines, saying he doesn't want to see my mother so soon after lying to her. In the driveway, I notice three unusual cars, one of which is my father's Mustang convertible. My parents aren't on friendly terms to say the least, so to have them both here in the house together seems unreal. Another of the cars belongs to Mr. Fazioli, the father of one of my high school friends. He's a loudmouthed Italian—funny as hell—who, like it or not, is the center of attention wherever he goes. I'm glad he's here. Maybe he'll break the tension between my parents. I don't know who owns the other car.

Once inside, the mystery of the third car is solved. Dr. Frei is here making an evening house call on my behalf. He's not a welcome sight, unless he's here to sign my discharge papers.

I settle into the family room, sitting as far away as I can from the shrink, reminding myself of my mother's promise to keep me out of the hospital. Her word means something to me.

She's never lied to me before and I don't expect her to start tonight. I can sit back and see how the clash of personalities plays out.

As always, Mr. Fazioli carries the room with jokes, laughter and a voluminous voice that overtakes the others. This impresses me. We've got two doctors, a distraught mother and an escaped mental patient, and yet it's good old Mr. Fazioli taking center stage.

But Dr. Frei is warming up for his own evening's agenda, which is to get my willful cooperation to return to the hospital. From across the room, he presents his plan using the familiar phrases, such as how I need to be "more stabilized" and that I'll only have to stay "a short time." It's a road I've been down before, and I know it won't be nearly as easy as he makes it sound. There'll be plenty of twists and turns and potholes, and for what? Where does the road end?

The problem right now is my parents and Mr. Fazioli. They're all standing around, nodding their agreement with Dr. Frei and expecting me to go along with his airtight reasoning. They think it sounds great—get stabilized and get out soon—no problem. How can I impress upon them the trap that is being set for me?

"It's a trap," I say.

But that only makes the situation worse because according to Dr. Frei traps are what paranoid people concoct in their minds.

Nods of agreement follow. It's clear that my bargaining power is wasting away to nothing, and my defenses are wearing thin again.

Mr. Fazioli jumps in to break the tension. Noting my state of inebriation, he puts forth his idea that alcohol is the crux of the problem. He thinks maybe I'm an alcoholic, and if I could quit drinking my problems would dissolve.

Though his reasoning sometimes falls short of the mark,

Mr. Fazioli is a man who's willing to put his money behind his words. He makes a deal with me. He says if I can go one full year without drinking a thing—no beer, no wine, no screwdrivers and no shots—he'll give me his Cadillac.

"Holy shit" I say, "that's a pretty good deal." I can't really see myself driving around in a Cadillac, not my style, but it might be nice for dates or for cruising up and down the Strip. If I don't like it after that, I can sell it along with my El Camino and buy something really nice, like a Porsche. The thought of it puts a smile on my face. Mr. Fazioli saves the day.

Now Dr. Frei is in a better position to deal with me. We turn back to the central topic of my being hospitalized. I relent, but under one condition, which is that I'll only be admitted to the open ward on the second floor. I can't tolerate another sentence in the locked ward, and I make this clear. "No fifth floor," I say, "no way."

Despite his reluctance, Dr. Frei goes along with my demand. Then the party breaks up and I'm on my way back to the hospital with my trash bag full of stuff.

True to his word, Dr. Frei reserves a bed for me on the second floor, but there's an attendant out in the hall watching me all night. I lie in bed thinking about the day's events and then drift into a scene of me driving around in Mr. Fazioli's Cadillac with a beautiful woman in the passenger seat. Even though I'm back where I started, I think the day's been a success. I had a few beers with a friend, my parents seemed to get along—thanks in part to me—and there's a Cadillac on layaway if I stay sober for a year. This makes it a pretty good day in my book. With these pleasant thoughts, I drift into a good night's sleep.

17

E ARLY the next morning Dr. Frei places an order to have me transferred up to the fifth floor, effective as soon as I'm awake. This wasn't part of our agreement, but I suppose in the twisted world of psychiatric doublespeak Dr. Frei can claim to be true to his word. After all, he did initially admit me on the second floor. The fact that my ass is hauled up to the locked ward the next morning is a minor detail.

Demoted and demoralized, back on the fifth floor, I walk around simmering with anger, ready to blow, but keeping things in check for the moment. I go to group therapy to keep the image of a compliant patient, but my heart isn't in it. Sitting here, looking around the room, I get more disgusted than ever. These people look like the most wretched losers on the planet—all of them brainwashed and too stupid to know it. A few of them sit comatose without uttering a word. One gaunt fellow is shaking like a paint mixer, but he's got a smile on his face and he says only positive things.

Early in the group, one of the patients yammers on about how nice the people are up here and how helpful the medications seem to be. This is followed by more pleasant testimonials from other patients. None of them show any inclination toward real emotion—no anger, no grief—just dull pleasantries and flatness. It's the kind of talk that makes me want to vomit. When it's my turn to speak, I can't contain it any longer.

"Every one of you needs a good kick in the ass," I say. I'm hoping for some kind of charged reaction from the group. But all I get is a concerned look from the social worker. She asks me to describe my feelings, which seems impossible to do without exploding in the process. Instead of exploding, I think the best thing is to leave the group.

As I get up to do so, the social worker says my name in a friendly way. She sounds concerned for me, which is not what I expect. For a couple of seconds I stand at the door unable to decide whether to stay or go. Looking back at the social worker, I see the concerned look again. It's enough to keep me in the room until group is over.

In the evening I'm allowed short visits with each parent, first my dad and then my mother. I tell my mother how mad I am and what I want to do with all the rage inside.

"I want to beat the shit out of somebody!" I say. "Anyone would do." I tell her I'd be better off dead, and if I just had the guts to jump out the window, the world would be a better place.

I'm not serious about killing myself—just venting—but to be on the safe side my mother reports the threat to the nurse's station, and they in turn put me on suicide watch for the next two days. That's what I get for venting.

Now a staff person approaches me every 15 minutes with pad and pen in hand, charting what I'm doing.

Day after day, the oppressiveness of the fifth floor takes its toll on me. It's a gradual shift in perspective where the other patients don't look so bizarre anymore. Most of them seem like wasted zombies, but what's so bad about that? Within a few days I stop arguing with the nurse about taking the drugs. I also ease up on demanding to go home or down to the second floor.

Normally mealtime is the most pleasant diversion, other than sleep, but meals on the fifth floor are a poor excuse for sustenance. The kitchen staff brings up a cartload of hot trays at mealtime, but the food is barely warm by the time we get it. The food on the trays looks like leftover slop for a herd of pigs. The patients aren't exactly pig-like, but watching some of them eat, with their drooling and their dyskinetic herky-jerky and food going all over the place, doesn't lend much in the way of dining ambience. I keep my head down and eat like a robot, trying to ignore anything disgusting in the periphery.

My compliant behavior is at last rewarded. After six days in the locked ward, Dr. Frei authorizes a transfer back down to the second floor. Once again, I seem to be on the right track.

Upon arriving on the second floor, my case manager invites me to attend group therapy. She's the same woman who gave me that concerned look up on the fifth floor, and I like her for that. Her name is Rhonda, and though she doesn't have much of a sense of humor she's caring and pretty to look at, especially her curvy figure, her dark sensuous eyes and her smooth skin. I want to make a good impression, so I generally go along with whatever she requests. It's too bad she doesn't ask me to give her a back rub or anything like that. Strictly professional is she.

I sit in group therapy, looking around at these unfamiliar people, and I'm nervous as hell. I wonder where the nerves are coming from. Maybe it has to do with this new lot of patients. Here the people are much more on the ball, and it feels threatening. I'm used to being the sharpest of the bunch up on the fifth floor. But these people could run circles around my feeble brain.

As we go around the room, patients talk about how they voluntarily checked themselves into this place. *They actually want to be here.* To me this seems like the most masochistic thing you could do. But the patients look almost content, like they're on vacation from all the stress of life. Who needs the Bahamas with people like this?

After a couple of group sessions, I start paying more attention to the voluntary patients, hoping their cheery outlook will rub off on me. To some extent the strategy works because a few people have said they like the changes they see in me. I'm not so sure. For one, I can't maintain a decent conversation for more than a few minutes. I sit and listen and understand fairly well, but I can't get into the flow. By the time I think of something good to say, the moment passes or someone else already said it.

To make matters worse Dr. Frei switches my medication again, getting rid of Prolixin, returning to Thorazine and starting another neuroleptic drug called Stelazine. He says this new combination will be better for my blood pressure. He doesn't seem to care much when I complain about the other side effects, such as turning into a dimwitted zombie. I'm also showing this strange habit of tapping my open hands together, as if they're two spiders bouncing off each other. When I ask the shrink what's causing this, he says he doesn't know whether it's the drugs or the underlying illness.

In addition to group therapy we have educational groups, a few of which involve presenters from the outside community. Among the topics are assertiveness training, forgiveness and gratitude and, the more rudimentary, social skills lessons. I sit and listen with a good amount of interest while the teaching is going on, but as soon as it's over I forget just about all that's been said. We also have arts and crafts and almost daily walks to the park over by the New River. On rare occasions there are escorted trips to the Galleria mall, which make me feel completely out of place. Being in a mental hospital doesn't instill much of an urge to shop.

When we aren't doing some type of group activity, I sometimes get individual attention from the staff. Most of these encounters are a welcome break from the boredom, but one of the social workers brings out the worst in me. She's an attractive blonde with a high-pitched, singsong voice and she's pleasant to look at, which is fine if it stops there. But her habit of overdramatizing everything like it's all a huge deal makes me tired. Worse yet is the tone she uses when she talks to me. It's like I'm an eight-year-old boy again. If there's anything that irritates me, it's when people talk down to me as though I'm a little kid. Part of my irritation is the fact that I feel like a child these days, with the drugs giving me the mental apparatus of a ball peen hammer, so I don't need to be reminded about it from the likes of this social worker. If I have to listen to her sympathetic voice for very long, my head may explode. To keep my frustration down, I tune her out and try to imagine her naked…and mute.

This brings up the matter of sex, a topic weighing heavily on my mind these days. Despite my enfeebled state, I still have a sex drive, frustrated as it is. Life would be easier if the drugs washed that away with everything else, but they don't. I'm not one of these sexual animals going around harassing women, and I don't go for masturbating in a mental ward, like Neil in Alabama. But with the boredom on high, and the days and weeks and months without sex, and me in my so-called sexual prime, I feel frustrated. Just about any woman with a pair of tits has my attention.

Weekends at the hospital are the most difficult time. With the staff down to a skeleton crew, there aren't any decent activities available. The TV blares nonstop in the day room with glazed patients sitting in front of it. Most patients on the second floor are out on passes with family members if they have any family around. I'm lucky enough to have mine involved, and by the second weekend since my escape Dr. Frei allows me go out on passes again.

The first of these occurs on Saturday, April 14th with my mother and sisters. It's Christine's 21st birthday and she's excited about it. At home I watch her open presents from everyone except me. I suppose I have a good excuse for not getting her anything, but I still feel bad about it. Later in the day, after being deposited back at the hospital, I pace up and down the hallway feeling bored and empty.

The next day I get another pass with my father. We spend most of the time working outside, washing and waxing his car and fixing a few of the sprinklers in his lawn. I don't have the energy to do the work, which slows down my father, probably making it less efficient than if he did everything himself. I also get nervous as hell for no reason I can explain. The more I think about it, the more nervous I get. I tell my dad about the nerves, and he can see that it's a pretty big deal. So, being a doctor and all, he decides to take immediate action. Never mind the fact that he's a gynecologist.

My father gives me a dose of something sedating called meprobamate, which works to calm me down for a while. But by the end of the pass, my nerves are firing away again. When my dad delivers me back to the hospital, he tells the charge nurse what he's done and says I should have another dose of the stuff soon. But since there's no order written for meprobamate, the nurse is none too pleased with my dad's course of action. She and my father argue over it and they both get pretty heated. My dad has to be escorted off the floor by an attendant.

After all the commotion, the nurse gives me something called Librium, which seems no different from the stuff my father gave me. It's the principle of the thing I guess.

Monday morning I'm back to the daily routine of groups and activities. I hope to be discharged by the end of the week or even sooner. The earliest estimate according to Rhonda is Wednesday. But even three more days feels like forever.

The anxiety I felt yesterday with my dad is back again. After morning group therapy is over, I pace the hallway with my headphones on, trying to shake off the nerves. The pacing and the music have the effect of rousing me into a state of anger, which if given a choice is better than nervousness. Sustained anger is something I haven't felt for a while. Mostly it's mellow here. In fact, it's so mellow that my anger is sure to be noticed.

Among the things to avoid are yelling, screaming, punching or destroying things, and I've got the sense to know better. All I do is tell the nurse how angry I feel, how I want to leave, and how I *want* to tear the place apart. I'm just venting my frustrations, being careful not to produce another explosion. I want to see if the nurse can help me or at least direct me to someone who can.

But her idea of help is not what I had in mind. The nurse says she wants me transferred back up to the locked ward.

"Wait a minute," I say. "Hold on." I accuse her of overreacting, and I try to take back what I said, explaining the difference between wanting to break things and actually breaking them. But it's not coming out clearly enough. The nurse calls for attendants to escort me back to the fifth floor.

This puts me over the edge. Instantly I'm enraged, ready to fire away at anyone. "Fuck you!" I say to the nurse. "Fuck all of you!" to the rest of the staff.

The attendants wrap my arms behind my back and wrestle me into the elevator. Once we get to the top floor, they wrestle me down the hall while I kick and flail around, using my head as a weapon. I'm an easy catch for them. They drag me into the seclusion room and cuff me diagonally in two-point restraints.

Locked up and restrained, I remain a fuming animal, energized by the power of focused anger. This is my new reality, and it feels far more real than the pathetic lamb I've been over the past two weeks. All that saccharin sweetness makes me want to puke now. No more kissing the asses of these mindless drones.

Early Tuesday morning a nurse comes in to give me my scheduled battery of drugs. She presents them on a little tray with a cup of juice to mask the horrible taste. I tell her she's wasting her time. Then I grab the tray and throw it across the room with the pills and liquid flying off in different directions. The size of the mess makes me think they've added more drugs.

This nurse isn't a mean person, and she tries to be civil about the whole ordeal. Rather than go directly for the syringe, she calls my father and enlists him to pressure me into taking the drugs.

The voice of reason hasn't completely left me. I'm willing to listen to my dad, but he's not enough to make me back down. After the phone call, I tell the nurse to read the list of drugs and explain what each is supposedly for.

In the spirit of cooperation, she does what I ask. The list is longer than I remember. Now there's Benadryl and an unfamiliar drug, Tranxene, to go along with the Stelazine, Thorazine and Cogentin. Plus, I now have the option of Librium or sodium amytal as emergency drugs in case of a total meltdown. The list reads like a cocktail menu from hell. But, just to assuage my father and the nurse, I agree to take this new medication Tranxene but nothing else.

Then I ask for something you'd think I have a reasonable chance of getting. I ask for my Walkman. I say it's necessary to help me relax and fight off the boredom of seclusion. But the request is denied. Apparently Dr. Frei sees a connection between my listening to the radio and my latest episode. He figures the radio is triggering me into hostility and possibly feeding the delusions. So he keeps it under lock and key for the time, which makes me furious.

After some fitful hours of sleep I awaken Wednesday morning, still in seclusion although not restrained and still angry, threatening to kill anyone who forces the drugs on me. I pace back and forth in the windowless room like a rabid hyena, yelling and spitting.

I'm duly rewarded for my behavior with the addition of four-point restraints and dual shots of sodium amytal and Thorazine. At lunchtime, with my left hand free, I take the food tray and throw it against the wall. I figure there isn't anything good on there anyway.

As for the process of seclusion, restraints and shots, there isn't much new variety here. It's the same thing from one institution to another in terms of dealing with non-compliant behavior. The only new twist here is that they call it the *quiet room*, as if this is how you're supposed to get once you're locked in.

I take issue with the title, yelling to anyone who can hear, "This ain't no fucking quiet room!" Then I spit until there's no spit left.

18

A FTER two solid days of being locked up, the whole thing gets old. As the yelling and other antics subside, I reduce myself to pleading and begging to be let out. It's always the same set of conditions to gain my release: take the drugs and behave in an appropriate manner. Call me a slow learner, but finally I realize there's no other way but to submit.

By the time it's over, after four and a half days of carrying on and refusing the drugs, my butt is as sore as an open wound from all the shots. To show what a compassionate guy he is, Dr. Frei orders *warm soaks* for my bottom. So now I'm entitled to the luxury of having a staff person come to my bed at regular intervals to lay a hot, wet towel across my suffering ass.

Out of seclusion, but still in the locked ward, I drift back to being a docile lamb. It's not like I have much choice in the matter. The lamb is their creation.

One of the things I do when my ass isn't throbbing in pain is sit in the day room and look out the window at the old mansion across the street. From this high perch, I can see the huge structure and much of the landscape surrounding it. It has an imposing wall built around it to keep out the riff-raff and an intricate garden behind the wall with vines and tropical greenery. The mansion was built in an ornate Spanish style, and it looks like a compound for some Third World despot hiding from society. It also looks vacant.

I scan for signs of human life and find nothing. But then I see a couple of workmen going into the place with tools and a ladder. The thought occurs to me that they're preparing the place for me, that I'll be granted the homestead in compensation for all my troubles. Maybe it's God's way of saying that I passed the test after all. The only drawback would be the view of the wacko ward across the street.

Even though I see the absurdity and the grandiosity of my thinking, I still want to believe it's true. My thoughts go back and forth between cursing myself for holding out hope and then hoping once more that it might be true.

On the second evening out of seclusion, my father visits. It's the first time I've seen him in nearly a week, during which time he received daily updates about my condition from Dr. Frei. Since the news was rarely good, my father has grown frustrated. When he arrives we talk about the tired monotony of going from hospital to hospital and now, back and forth between the second and fifth floor. Then he says something that really gets to me. He says, "You know this is costing me a lot of money. You've got to get well soon."

The statement has me dumbfounded. I don't know what to say. It hasn't occurred to me how much my old man is shelling out to keep me here. Even though it's mostly covered by insurance, the weekly co-pay is over $400. But then I think about what an insensitive bastard he is to make that kind of remark. It almost sounds like a threat. Does he think I'm enjoying myself here, idling away my time like it's the fucking Ritz Carlton?

And is that the only reason he wants me to get better, so I'm not such a drain on his bank balance? The weight of it sinks in, and I feel as helpless as if I were in four-point restraints.

After he's gone, my helpless feeling is replaced by renewed anger toward the man. I could easily explode. But instead, I go to a couple of social workers to talk about it, thus avoiding my being strapped to a bed.

The next day I'm transferred again down to the open ward, but to be safe the staff keeps the exit doors at the ends of the hallway locked.

Normally, on the open unit we all go down to the ground floor cafeteria for meals, and there we can choose whatever we want to eat. It's something I look forward to, especially after the slop I've been eating up on the locked ward. It's also kind of nice sitting with staff and patients from other floors who have cafeteria privileges.

There's this girl on the adolescent unit who's interested in me. She wrote me a love letter a couple of weeks ago, which I read over and over again, each time fantasizing about how great it would be to escape from this place with her by my side. Together we could make a break for the beach, taking side streets to keep clear of the cops. It would be easy to evade the police on foot, and she would see what a brave guy I am. We could have our first French kiss while hiding out in dense bushes near a canal, or under a tarp on someone's sailboat. Once at the beach, we'd be filled with passionate longing. If the waves aren't too big, we could swim out to a sand bar and sex it up right there. My dick gets hard just thinking about it. Or we could walk down to Birch State Park and find a secluded picnic table or a cabin with bunk beds. I go over the possibilities every time I read the letter.

But the staff is on to me. They know about my romantic interest on the adolescent unit, and they aren't taking any chances with me down in the cafeteria, not while she's there. Instead, I have to sit alone in the day room and wait for a lunch tray to be delivered.

With a little coaxing, I'm able to talk a social worker into letting me go down there to get a drink at the soda fountain. He walks me to the lunch line where I fill two cups, all the while looking around for the girl from the fourth floor. She isn't here yet, or maybe she already left. I want to hang out a little longer but the social worker won't let me. Back I go to eat and drink in solitude.

In the evening, while visiting with my mother, I tell her what a terrible joke this is turning out to be. I tell her I don't have any problems, except for those inflicted on me by the institution. And I tell her that I want to leave this place tomorrow morning.

Fearing the worst, my mother goes to the nurses' station with this latest information, and they in turn have me transferred back up to the fifth floor.

After a restless night of sleeping and battling with the sheets, I awaken angry and frustrated. By 9 A.M. I'm confined once again to the so-called quiet room. Extra medication is given, and I'm smart enough this time not to refuse it. I take it orally because my ass is still sore from the last quiet room adventure. By ten o'clock I'm asleep again. As always, a sleeping patient is a good patient.

Groggy-eyed and exhausted, I awaken just in time for lunch. I take my meal without complaint. Good behavior wins me a ticket out of seclusion shortly thereafter.

My father is set to arrive for an evening visit, but I'm in no mood to see him. His comment from last time is still weighing heavily on my mind. I can't shake the thought of beating him senseless.

Up and down the hall I pace, waiting for my father, and I can feel the anger rising. He meets me at the nurses' station and together we go to my room. He says I should sit down, but I don't feel like sitting. I have nothing good to say. So I stand by the door silently, trying to fend off my anger. Dad is standing across from me and he says something. I don't know what he says, but it triggers the animal in me. I clench my right fist and hammer it into his face, connecting on the left side of his mouth.

He backs out of the room, cupping his bloody mouth, and returns to the nurses' station. He tells the charge nurse what his son just did and then leaves the hospital, loose tooth and all. He's dripping blood all over the front of his shirt as he drives off.

A nurse comes into my room armed with two male attendants, and she gives me an unscheduled dose of Thorazine. I take it without protest. Then I march myself over to the seclusion room and sit on the bed. No one said I have to be here—it just seems the best thing to do. The nurse asks if I want to talk about the incident.

"No, I don't want to talk about anything."

So she leaves.

Alone I sit, wracked with guilt, thinking about the terrible thing I just did. This has to be a new low point—assaulting my old man. What kind of crazed animal does that? Up to now, I could make the case that every act of aggression I ever committed was in self-defense. But now I bloodied my own father without provocation, except for a few insensitive remarks. And he didn't even try to fight back. That makes it even more pitiful. At least if he fought back I could say that he's been storing up a lot of hostility for me, and all I did was release it. The more I think about it, the weaker my excuses seem. I'm such a fucking loser. I have to make some changes.

19

NOTING my slow rate of progress and my continued risk for flight, the staff arranges a court hearing to have my involuntary status lengthened by another month. The hearing is held on April 30th, and it includes a public defender, a general master of the courts, Dr. Frei, my mother and Rhonda to handle the details. I'm not sure how to conduct myself during the meeting but it hardly matters. The outcome seems nonnegotiable from the start. I could act like a rabid chimp in a cage, or I could be the model of mental stability, and the result would be the same — 30 days mandated placement, without passes. The only loophole here is that the psychiatrist has the power to override the order and let me out early. I'm smart enough not to count on that happening.

This meeting is a legal formality of the larger system with its own cryptic language, and it reaffirms my role as a powerless pawn. It's during this meeting that the combined issues of *insight* and *judgment* are brought to the foreground. Normally you'd think the term insight means something deep, like self-knowledge regarding the nature of your personality. According to Freud and others, insight is an essential component of mental health. To be well and to function in a healthy way, you need to know about the psychic forces determining your personality, so the theory goes. Never mind the fact that your insight has to match their theory of how you function.

Here too in the psychiatric wards of 1984, insight is considered important for recovery. But the hospital definition doesn't have the depth of meaning that Freud's term had. In this context, insight means little more than accepting that you have a mental illness requiring proper medical treatment. That's it. It's like the drunk who gets up in front of a bunch of fellow drunks and says, "Hello my name is Ted, and I'm an alcoholic." Thus Ted has insight, which is the hallmark first ingredient to lasting sobriety. Substitute the diagnosis, schizophrenic for alcoholic, and there you have it. How proud I think the staff would be if I could just say it and get it over with! That would be their little victory over my soul. Then I'd have insight in their eyes and be on the road to recovery, except for the fact that schizophrenics never really recover. Their best hope is to go into remission.

The second issue is judgment, which is a bigger nut to crack. It has to do with whether you've got the reasoning power and enough behavioral control to live out in the world without the need for supervision. According to the staff and mainstream psychiatry, the term also means that you realize you must take your medication to keep your illness under control. It's akin to the diabetic who knows he has to take insulin to keep living. That's exhibiting good judgment. Psychiatrists would like you to believe mental illness is no different.

Like modern crusaders, pharmaceutical companies spend many millions of dollars in a worldwide campaign to get their message of drug dependency across to psychiatrists and the lay public. Meanwhile, the science in their position is lacking. Drug company research is biased in their favor, and psychiatrists are notoriously bad scientists. As a result, the issue of whether patients really benefit from drug treatment over the long haul has not been answered in a credible way.

Dr. Frei is correct in the meeting when he says I lack insight and judgment, as per his definitions. I don't feel the slightest inclination to stand up and proclaim that I have a brain disease or a chemical imbalance, nor do I think I need his drugs to maintain mental stability. By adopting Dr. Frei's brand of insight and judgment, I would be consigning my brain to the medical establishment. From there, it could easily be a one-way trip into psychiatric never-never land.

On the fifth floor, patients come and go with no regularity. Most of them are what you'd call hard-core patients destined to spend long periods in state hospitals, if they haven't been there already.

One day a female patient tells me a horror story about one of the state mental hospitals. She says she was raped repeatedly by a couple of male attendants. The rapes took place during the night shift in a locked stairwell. At first she screamed, but this only got her slapped around and knocked against a concrete wall. She says she tried to report it, but no one believed her, and the guys who raped her threatened to kill her if she opened her mouth again. So she took the abuse night after night until she got transferred out. She says the fifth floor of the Fort Lauderdale Hospital is a blessing, and to her it surely is.

At about this time I get assigned a new roommate who annoys the hell out of me. He talks to himself all hours day and night about nonsense as far as I can tell. He also flicks the lights on and off throughout the night, which interrupts any brief segment of sleep I might get. I want to go over to his bed and smack his face with the heel of my shoe, but I think better of it. After voicing my complaints, the guy is transferred to another room. But it doesn't matter anyway because I'm headed back down to the second floor.

In my newly assigned room, my father visits me for the first time since I punched him in the face. It's been over a week and he looks pretty well healed, which is good. He's also friendly, saying nothing about the incident or what led up to it, which is also good. I hope he's not waiting for me to bring it up because that's the last thing I want to talk about. I'm still ashamed about hitting him, but I don't feel the need to apologize. He could just as well apologize to me, and maybe then I'll say that I'm sorry for the way I reacted.

As it turns out, neither of us would bring up the incident on this day, nor any other day for years to come. Instead, we keep to the safe conversational territory of cars and the work he plans to do on his Mustang. So things are back to normal again between my father and me. Put stitches over an open wound and carry on. That's how we do it.

The next couple of days are a difficult affair. One night I stay up for hours filled with strange thoughts about werewolves howling at the full Moon. Normally such thoughts wouldn't bother me, but now I'm starting to see them as a problem. It's like my mind is this wild animal that can't be tamed, and the rest of me has to go along for the ride. Some trips are good and some are hellish, as if stripped from the pages of Dante's Inferno. It's a lonely thing to have such thoughts, especially in the middle of the night.

To get some measure of comfort and understanding, I go to the nurses' station. For a few minutes the night nurse is pleasant and all, but then she gets out the Thorazine and says it should do the trick. The message I get is that comforting words are fine, but it's the drugs that really count. For the first time, I start thinking that maybe I need the drugs after all. The thought of it depresses the hell out of me.

The next day I'm a mess. I go back and forth between tears and anger, and I'm constantly seeking comfort from the staff. I have to excuse myself from group when I think I might say something outlandish. In response, my medication is increased, which helps thrust out the mental images and further dulls my brain.

After dinner, my mother arrives in my room and sees that I'm a crying, desperate mess. Amidst the tears, I confess my fear that I'll never be able to live a normal life again. "It'll be one goddamn hospital after another," I say.

She doesn't agree or disagree, but tries to support me as best she can.

Even with increased medication the sleepless nights continue. Always there to help, Dr. Frei puts in an order for Halcion, which I can attest is one potent sleeping aid. It's also highly addictive. Over the course of about a week, I come to rely on the drug almost like an addict. Halcion is the god of dreamless sleep.

Realizing I'm a tough case to crack, Dr. Frei has me undergo a consultation with another shrink, and together they came up with the false idea that I might be suffering from manic depression, also known as bipolar disorder. Dr. Frei says I show signs of mood swings in which, for two or three days, I'm depressed to the point of refusing to get out of bed. Then, at other times, I walk around in pretty good spirits with an occasional grandiose thought or two. At such times I have the racing thoughts where it's hard for me to keep up with the scattered maze of ideas. So my symptoms might be due to a mood disorder rather than the psychotic illness Dr. Frei has already pegged me with. As a kind of test for this new theory, he decides to add lithium—trade name Eskalith—to the current battery of drugs I'm already on.

In 1984 lithium is gaining popularity as the drug of choice

for manic depression. Although it's considered a drug, it's also a naturally occurring element, which lends it a kind of appeal, like you're taking something natural and safe, and it's actually something already found in the human body. But I'm not convinced that this is a strong selling point. Just because a thing is found in the *Periodic Table of Elements* and is detected in humans doesn't make it therapeutic. Consider mercury or lead, both of which are found in the body and neither of which is exactly conducive to bodily functioning. Like mercury and lead, lithium is also toxic when given in sufficient doses. There are people who swear by lithium treatment for the management of their mood disorder, but there's probably an even greater number who've tried it and found it not only unhelpful but also far too obnoxious to tolerate—worse than the mood disturbance itself.

The appeal of lithium as a treatment choice during my hospitalization brings up the point about a patient's treatment options being dependent on the time period in which the person is treated. That is to say, *how* you're treated is contingent upon *when* you're treated. For example, let's say I was treated in 1948 instead of 1984. Back then I might've been the recipient of a frontal lobotomy.

Basically this procedure involves the use of a metal probe, not unlike an ice pick, which is inserted just above the eyeball, through the socket, taking special care not to poke the eyeball itself. Using the probe, the surgeon feels around for the fissure dividing the frontal from the parietal lobe of the brain. Once the fissure is found, he pokes the probe up until it touches the skull. From there it's just a matter of sweeping it back and forth like a windshield wiper, clearing away all the unwanted neural connections. The process is then repeated for the other side.

With both sides properly severed and the probe removed, the patient is considered cured, assuming the surgeon didn't botch it. The patient is now free of any trouble from that pesky frontal lobe. But to say that he's a changed man is a gross understatement. He has hardly a trace of creativity or spontaneity left, and his achievement drive is almost nonexistent. His abstract reasoning is also pretty well shot. But, on the positive side, at least he'll save money on those expensive opera tickets, and he won't have to waste time on that Impressionist art exhibit at the local museum. Apple juice and the Weather Channel will suit him just fine.

Lobotomies fell out of fashion with American psychiatrists in the mid-1950's, when they discovered they could get the same mind-stripping results from the drug Thorazine. But who knows? The lobotomy might make a comeback. To be on the safe side, I'd watch out for psychiatrists walking around with ice picks. Actually, with modern technology, they'd be more likely to use lasers and call it something sophisticated and benign, like Corrective Neural Reprogramming, or CNR for short.

I can see two psychiatrists chatting about the procedure over lunch. One says, "Hey, how about that tough patient in 204? You think he's ready for CNR?"

To which the other psychiatrist says, "I don't know. What insurance does he have?"

Another therapeutic procedure I miss out on is shock treatment, or electroconvulsive therapy (ECT), which has gone through ebbs and flows in popularity since the late 1930's. In this modality, electrodes are positioned at the sides of the head. It used to be the whole head that was shocked, but now they mostly limit it to the right hemisphere, which I guess is the more disposable part of the brain in our society. Before administering the electric current, the patient is rendered unconscious by an anesthesiologist, due to the high voltage blast about to take place. The result of the shock is a convulsion, similar to a grand mal seizure, which destroys nerve cells in the affected brain regions. Memory loss is the most obvious result, but there may be other subtle effects as well, like emotional dulling.

ECT is given most often to those suffering from severe and chronic depression, and many patients do report feeling better, at least in the week or so following the procedure. Maybe it's because they can't remember the stuff that made them feel so bad.

After starting me on lithium Dr. Frei again decides to take me off Thorazine, given the havoc it causes with my blood pressure. He keeps the Stelazine in place, but also adds a different neuroleptic drug to the mix. This one is called Trilafon. The Cogentin is kept in place to combat side effects, and I get sodium amytal, Librium and Halcion as standard backup options.

This game of musical chairs with medication is common psychiatric practice, which often takes place behind the scenes with little or no discussion with the patient. That's how it is with me. Consent is not an issue, and I'm not warned of the drugs' potential side effects.

One of the well-known side effects of these drugs is a permanently disabling muscle disorder, known as tardive dyskinesia, or TD. It's characterized by odd repetitive movements, like the twisting and smacking of the tongue, strange facial grimaces and wringing of the hands, as if the person is shaking off water after washing dishes. There's also a stiff wooden gait that goes with it. It's like getting a case of brain damaging Parkinson's disease, but the damage is caused by the drugs. And, Like Parkinson's, the condition is irreversible.

I don't realize I'm at risk for getting TD, but there are patients on the fifth floor who have it pretty bad. I doubt they were given any warning about the risk, and they probably don't even know how they got it. Psychiatrists often cover up the severity of the condition and downplay your chances of getting it.

Later in life, I would observe a psychiatrist telling a patient that her TD symptoms are part of the schizophrenia and not the result of drug treatment. It's a convenient little reversal of facts, you might say. It's no exaggeration to say that Dr. Frei is playing Russian roulette with TD, knowing there's a chance I could get it from the stuff he's giving me. But again this is standard practice, with TD serving as an acceptable risk for the greater good.

20

THE 11th of May is a pivotal day for me. As long as I keep my emotions under control, I'm allowed limited privileges to listen to my Walkman. On this day I pace up and down the hall with headphones on, thinking about how long I've been here and conversely how long I've gone without seeing friends and doing the things in life I want to do. I tally it up and figure I've been here nine weeks, which is a startling amount of time. I'm no better now than the day I first set foot in this place and maybe even worse.

Pondering the situation brings back a level of indignation, which I guess is visible from the way I'm walking. One of the nurses comes over and asks me to relinquish the radio. I fuss about it but give it up after a half-hearted argument.

With no groups scheduled and nothing to do I call my mother, not realizing a staff person is within earshot of my voice. This is unfortunate because during the conversation I tell my mother that I feel like a modern day Jesus, destined to be persecuted for the rest of my life. I tell her I'm not sick at all, just misunderstood as was Christ, and the whole staff is bent on crucifying me.

After the phone call I realize the damage is done. There's a nurse looking at me while she dials up Dr. Frei. The inevitable outcome will surely be more drugs and a trip back up to the locked ward. But not if I can help it.

I tell the nurse that I'm tired and need to lie down as I head in the direction of my room. Passing the room, I quicken my pace to the end of the hallway and down the unlocked stairwell. Once outside, I break into a sprint westward on Las Olas to the familiar convenience store. It's the same place where I called Bill from five weeks ago. It would be too obvious to call him again—first place they'd search—so I go into the store to think over my options.

Trying not to be conspicuous, I browse the aisles and look over the assortment of snack items and emergency toiletries. I have a few dollars on me and, given the amount of time I'm spending here dawdling around the place, I think it's a good idea to buy something. It's about 10 A.M. and I'm not hungry in the slightest, but something to drink would be nice. I gaze over the assortment of juices, milk, sodas and beer, lingering a little longer at the beer. No, that's not a good idea and at ten o'clock in the morning, no less. That's the last thing I should have. Only a true alcoholic drinks before noon.

But then I have a little argument with myself, the outcome of which is that a beer is the perfect choice. It's a symbolic *fuck you* to Fort Lauderdale Hospital and to Dr. Frei and to the whole system holding me captive. Having a beer is my way of telling them they haven't got me yet, despite their best efforts.

So I purchase a cold can of Busch, which is the cheapest option, save for the unpalatable stuff. The cashier puts it in a can-size brown paper bag, like the way bums have their beverages. I check for anyone suspicious, then walk around to the back alley behind the store to drink it.

Despite the fact that it cost me Mr. Fazioli's Cadillac, which I don't deserve anyway, the cold beer goes down smooth. After it's done, I urinate on the side of a dumpster, re-pack and head east on Las Olas, toward the beach. Maybe I can clear my head with the sounds of the waves and the seagulls and all. And it won't hurt to keep my eyes open for early rising bikinis.

I cross the drawbridge over the Intracoastal Waterway and head north on A1A, walking up the ocean side of the street. This stretch of road is the Strip, of spring break fame, with an assortment of hotels, shops and bars on the western side of the street and the beach and the Atlantic Ocean on the east. If it's sunny, you can always count on seeing a wide mix of people here. There are homeless misfits, teenage punks, silicon-implanted beauties, gay men in Speedo's, Cubans, Haitians, Yankee retirees in Bermuda shorts and rich Italians cruising up and down in gaudy convertibles. Add one escaped mental patient to the list.

I suppose the closest I come to any of these groupings is a homeless misfit, hoping for invisibility. Being homeless, though, is a culture in itself and not one I care to join. I still have a home and a family, and I'd like to go back despite what the mental health community says.

It's tough to know what to do. Other than my current attire, I've got nothing, not even a garbage bag with clothes and personal items. After thinking the situation over, I come up with the only plan that makes sense—to try convincing my mother again to let me stay home, where I swear I won't be a problem. That's what I set out to do.

Maintaining a northward course, I walk alongside Birch State Park and through Galt Ocean Mile. So far, I've walked about five miles at a slow but steady pace. It's exhausting in the midday heat, with the soles of my feet burning in hot sneakers and my gait clumsy in the fog of neuroleptics. By the time I approach Lauderdale-by-the-Sea, I'm drenched with sweat but determined to go on without a break. At the same awkward pace, I head west on Commercial Boulevard over the draw-bridge and onto Bayview Drive.

Approaching my house, I get a sunken feeling in my chest. Two police cars and an ambulance are parked in the driveway awaiting my arrival. The scene shouldn't be a surprise by now, but it's a startling thing anyway. I think of running, but I doubt I'd get very far. I throw my hands up in the air. "You got me," I say. For now I'll play by their rules.

To demonstrate total compliance, I'm the picture of calm as a cop escorts me to the ambulance. Maybe the walk and the beer and the salty air did me some good. And maybe I've suc-cessfully sweated out half the neuroleptics circulating in my body.

In the ambulance I decline the offer to lie in bed for the trip back to the hospital. I want to sit up and look out the window. Who knows when I'll get another drive?

We travel back the same route that Danny, Peter and I took on the last day of high school, passing the same spot we drove on Victoria Park Road. Here's the place where at least two lives changed in irrevocable ways. Though unlikely, I wonder if this is the same ambulance that carted off Lois' unconscious body, leaving her bicycle behind. Wouldn't that be poetic jus-tice or sinister irony, or whatever you want to call the balanc-ing forces of nature?

My thoughts swing back and forth between that terrible day and today's ambulance-ride-one-way-ticket back up to the locked ward. For the first time, I'm able to think about Lois without flinching or constructing excuses for the way I acted that day. And, for the first time, I have a hint of compassion for myself and for the way things turned out. I want the ride to last a long time so I can sit with these thoughts. But before you could get out the words *involuntary commitment*, we're back on site, pulling up to the side door.

✳

When I arrive on the fifth floor I find the sum total of my belongings, minus the Walkman, on my newly assigned bed. I don't feel like unpacking, nor do I want to spend time chatting with the staff or patients. Instead I want to be left alone, so I ask if I can occupy the seclusion room with the door unlocked.

It's amazing what a difference there is between being in seclusion voluntarily, versus being forced in here against your will for an unknown duration. The first can serve as a valuable time for figuring things out, while the second can make you go nuts. This time in the so-called quiet room I'm actually quiet, lying in bed motionless yet awake, trying not to move a single muscle, as if to move would be an internal assault. My breathing slows to a relaxed rhythm.

Thoughts drift back to childhood, around the age of eight or nine. Phil and I were watching a Dr. Seuss cartoon together. The story was both simple and profound, and by the time it was over we were inspired to take action. It was about these two human-like creatures called *Zax* (with *Zak* as the singular) who were noted for their stubbornness. They traveled alone toward each other from opposite lands, and their paths crossed in an isolated wilderness. Like the story of Oedipus, who killed his father when their paths crossed, these two Zax were not of a mind to give way and let the other pass. But unlike the ancient Greeks, they weren't violent, just stubborn as hell. So they stood there facing each other motionless, neither giving way. This went on a long time.

Others took note of the two still figures, but no one was able to break the standoff. Animals came and went and seasons passed with the jackass Zax still facing off. The lack of interference by the others was nearly as impressive as the standoff itself. Roads were built around the two beings, then a town, and eventually a full-fledged urban sprawl encompassed them.

I forget how the story resolved itself. There may have been some moral about stubbornness and how you can waste away your life with it, but that escapes me now.

For Phil and me, the most impressive thing was the stand-off and the frozen stillness, like stopping time itself. So we decided to *make like Zax* with our own added twist. Rather than standing on the ground face-to-face, we opted to perch ourselves shoulder-to-shoulder on top of the chain-linked fence at the side of my house. To keep our balance, we tied a long rope to the trunk of a palm tree about 30 feet away, making sure the two rope ends were long enough to reach the fence. Then we stood atop the fence, each with a taut rope in hand, facing the street.

It was a pretty original pastime, as far as I can tell—kind of like water skiing, at least in terms of the rope and the balance. Cars, squirrels and birds passed by without incident. A few neighbors observed the curious ritual and must've thought we were deranged when we announced we were "playing Zax," like it's the natural thing for kids to do. My mother also considered the game strange, but since we weren't destroying anything or making a lot of racket, she consented.

We might've played this game five or ten times—I don't recall. What I do remember is the last time we did it. It rained like hell that day, soaking us to the bone. At first we thought we should get down out of the rain, but in the spirit of Zax we agreed to stay with it. We counted the seconds between the lightning and the thunder. The strikes weren't really close, but just to be sure Phil said it was bad to stand the way we were, under a tree, when there's lightning around, forgetting for the moment that we were also perched on a goddamn metal fence. So he said we should move down the fence closer to the house where we could get clear of the tree. That's what we did.

As we transferred ourselves down the fence, Phil stepped onto the top of the gate without thinking. The gate was un-

latched and it swung open with the force of Phil's weight. He
went down and struck his right arm on the fence post as he fell
to the ground shrieking in agony. I jumped down and looked at
his arm. It didn't take an orthopedist to see that it was broken
with the bone all skewed at a disgusting angle. I ran inside to
tell my mother so we could get Phil over to the hospital. But
Phil, no longer embodying the spirit of the Zax, ran down to
his house to tell his mother. Somehow the charm of being a
Zak wore off that day.

In the seclusion room, I consider my own Zak-like stubbornness. By this time I've escaped, or at least tried to escape,
a total of four times since this whole ordeal started. Every escape resulted in my being apprehended and brought back with
further restrictions on my freedom. I've also refused to take
the medication countless times, but again the staff had a way
of getting it into me, regardless of my consent. Like a Zak,
I'm wasting my life while civilization continues out there for
everyone else.

Then again, I'm not the only stubborn Zak in here. There's
also Dr. Frei with his tireless penchant for drugging me up and
keeping me here against my will. These facts are becoming
crystal clear. Another clear fact is that trying to undermine his
authority is self-destructive. It's also time consuming and, not
to forget, a waste of money. The old saying, "If you can't beat
'em, join 'em" comes to mind. I cringe at the thought of it.

I consider a frightening notion, which is that Dr. Frei owns
the facility and is housing me here as a source of income. It
seems to me that it's the money he cares about most. And maybe he's pumping the drugs to strip away my will, making me
look sicker than I really am. This is a horrifying possibility,
and I wonder if it's true.

Without the option of escape or refusing the drugs, what
else is there for me to do? I conclude that the only sensible
thing is to fire Dr. Frei and replace him with another shrink. It

sounds like a brilliant idea.

The next day I enlist the help of a nurse to draft a letter of intent to change doctors. We play around with the wording and eventually get it to where it sounds acceptable to both of us. In the letter, I request a transfer to Dr. Jones' care. There's been talk among patients that this shrink is less inclined to use a lot of drugs, and he seems to get his patients discharged quicker than the other psychiatrists. He sounds almost too good to be true.

Normally, a transfer from one shrink to another is the patient's right, as long as the patient is competent and of legal age. I figure it's as good as done once my letter goes through the proper channels. What I don't consider is the extent to which Dr. Frei has my parents wrapped around his spindly fingers. A series of phone calls are made between the doctors, my parents and the staff with the end decision being that a change of psychiatrist is not appropriate for me. A few days later, the same nurse who helped me with the letter gives me the news that my request was denied. Neither Dr. Frei nor my parents ever mention the ordeal.

I'm not ready to let the matter rest so easily. I go around to some of the patients and staff, telling them what I think of Dr. Frei, saying there's a conspiracy to keep me locked up and drugged up. After some probing, I find out how much money he's making by treating me, despite only seeing me an average of five minutes a day. It's a huge sum, considering the simplicity of his treatment. I figure he prefers seeing me all drugged up because it makes the visits shorter and more manageable.

After about a week of pursuing this course of thought, with nothing to show for it, I write the whole thing off as a distraction. I put the matter aside and begrudgingly accept Dr. Frei's agenda for me. The full reality of my situation sinks in. There is no escape, no refusal of drugs and no changing to a different shrink. These are the basic ground rules, and it's time I accept them. By the last week in May, I offer no visible resistance.

Meanwhile, a wave of depression sets in, especially during the nighttime hours. I can't shake the realization that my so-called friends are ignoring me. They're too busy to bother with me, doing their own thing, living productive lives. And what a downer it would be for them to come here and see me all laid up and pathetic like this. I have a recent letter from Phil describing the great things happening in Auburn and how he'll be glad to have me back up there soon. But this only adds to the gloom. It's like a carrot dangling in front of a rabbit, never close enough to eat.

At first it's just the hurt feeling over my friends neglecting me. But then, with the force of time ticking away, it turns into a feeling of betrayal. Hard as it is to admit, my friends are no more than the fair weather variety. My family keeps visiting on a regular basis. But if this goes on long enough, maybe they'll lose interest as well. It has to be tiring coming in here day after day, bringing milkshakes to a zombie on an emotional roller coaster. Who could blame them for giving up on me? Looking into the future, I can see visits tapering off, calls no longer being returned and no more milkshakes to break up the monotony of the hospital diet.

I think my grandparents might be the first to cut back their visits, then my father, and eventually my sisters would follow suit. This would leave only my mother making regular rounds. She too might have a breaking point, but that's a remote possibility. Something cataclysmic would need to happen for her to stop visiting, which I guess means that the milkshakes will keep coming indefinitely. How pathetic it would be, having only my mother as my connection to the outside world.

I picture family gatherings where the name of the forgotten lunatic, now locked up in a state asylum, never gets mentioned. If my mother talks about visiting me earlier in the week, another family member would step in and hush her by saying, "I thought we weren't going to talk about him anymore."

Such are my thoughts in the late hours when sleep won't come. In these small hours my mind has a way of taking a thing, usually a depressing thing, and following it to its final n^{th} degree unchecked. Nocturnal insomnia is prime time for disturbing thoughts to flourish.

When I can't take it anymore, I get up and ask the nurse for that magic little Halcion tablet, which usually does the trick. By mid-morning my thoughts are decidedly more pleasant, with hopeful rationalizations about how things will turn out for the best. Then after the late local news on TV, lying in bed, the whole dreaded cycle returns.

21

THIS insomnia might be an effort on the part of my unconscious to give me a sort of wake-up call, and to some degree it's successful. One day a social worker asks, "Why don't you get your act together?" This antagonizing question plays on and on late at night in my brain, as if nothing else in the world exists but the dark and the question. Added to the mix is my father's plea for me to get well because, after all, I'm costing him a lot of money. The meter's still running. And then there's the blonde social worker pitying me with her babying, singsong voice. All of these voices conspire to cut me down at the knees. I have to find a way to shake them.

What emerges in the midst of these awful sanctions is the advice of Arthur from Imperial Point, telling me to walk it off. "Walk tall and proud," he says, as I reconstruct the scene in my mind. Maybe there's some wisdom in his words after all, which I haven't detected until now. Regardless, his advice is better than the crap I've been thinking about, and it's worth a try to get back on track.

By morning I've made a pact to use my spare time to walk—not just mindless pacing but deliberate walking. "Tall and proud," I say to myself.

It seems like the easiest thing once I set my mind to it. The first thing I notice is the calming effect it has on me, as if my nerves, previously all locked up, now have a release valve. A few days of deliberate walking and my thoughts take on a new focus. I see my father's words about my needing to get well in a different light. Despite his intent, whatever it was, I now interpret it as a call to rally my resources. It's almost like he's giving me a vote of confidence, as if I have power and choice in the matter. I recast his words into something like, "Son, you have the power to bring yourself out of this."

I've heard it said that the most healing words you'll ever hear are the words coming from within you. And, conversely, the most damaging words are your own damning self-statements. This is how it seems to me. Little by little, pacing up and down the hall, the balance shifts to healing words coming from within rather than self-recrimination.

My change in demeanor is apparent to the staff, as evidenced by increased privileges. The first of these granted is the right to climb up and down the western stairwell, which provides exercise and a break from the stupor of the fifth floor. Of course the door leading outside is locked. Next comes increased time using my Walkman and, finally, the right to spend a few hours each day on the second floor as prelude to a full transfer. This is set to occur on the 1st of June.

A couple of days before my transfer, another court hearing is held. Noting my apparent progress and lack of psychotic symptoms, Dr. Frei and the staff agree to a tentative discharge in the middle of June.

While the meeting is in session I pace up and down the hall, trying not to invest a lot of hope in the outcome. When it's over, Rhonda gives me the news.

"Thanks," I say, continuing to pace.

But then she stops me asking why I'm not more enthusiastic.

It's because I doubt the credibility of anything said in such meetings. They can change their minds in a split second. "I'll believe it when I see it."

Pacing is an activity that gets noticed in a psychiatric facility. The repetitive act conjures up the image of someone plagued with agitation, or at worst the person is responding to some sort of *command delusion*. This is a type of grandiose or ominous thought process in which, for example, the afflicted person might think the world would end if the pacing stopped. There's also the social aspect of pacing, which is to say there's no social interaction at all, and that's a bad sign to the staff. The idea of walking for therapeutic benefit doesn't seem valid to them. So at times during my walking, a nurse or a social worker stops me to inquire about my state of mind. Since I had likened myself to a modern day Christ three or four weeks ago, the staff wonders whether I still feel that way now. The bold inquirer asks, "Do you still think you're Jesus Christ?"

In no mood to play games, I say no and leave it at that. But the question is rhetorical, as if to confirm a long-standing belief about me being schizophrenic. It seems people afflicted with the condition go around proclaiming they're Christ or some notable prophet. You may find five or six Christs at any given facility across the country. Whenever they say it, the diagnosis is confirmed.

In the Eastern Hemisphere, such a person might proclaim to be Buddha, but that's not so outlandish because Buddhism espouses the idea that all beings have Buddha within. Mainstream Christianity doesn't allow for that kind of kinship with Christ, save for the tired act of communion. Maybe the Buddhists and the schizophrenics have it right after all. Perhaps we all have the essence of Christ within us, obscured and distorted as it may be.

To say such a thing at Fort Lauderdale Hospital is dangerous. For this type of thinking, they crank up the drugs and they tack on more days. By now, at last, I know better. The best thing is to keep walking the hall with a pleasant face for all to see—to be the glazed doughnut that I am, and to never say anything controversial.

It's misleading to say that I don't socialize. In fact, I get along pretty well with staff and fellow patients, striving as ever to be pleasant and agreeable.

One of the more colorful characters is a male patient of about 35 with the last name Rockoff. I'm not sure if that's his real name, but it's what he goes by and it fits. He speaks in a rapid, theatrical way and dresses in formal attire, usually with pressed Oxford shirts and shiny wing-tipped shoes. You couldn't miss him if you try, and most of us try.

The mission that preoccupies Mr. Rockoff above all others is the conquest of women, and he thinks he has it down to science. One day a group of us patients are sitting in the day room in which Mr. Rockoff is taking center stage. He's presenting the best pickup lines for any situation a guy might find himself in. To humor him, we throw out possible social scenarios, and he gives a line suited to the occasion. His chief reference is a book with a name like *A Hundred Foolproof Ways to Pick up Women*. But I doubt the author had in mind a fool the likes of Mr. Rockoff. Here in the day room, with equal parts male and female present, our resident self-proclaimed Don Juan works the audience, acting out his lines, getting rejected all over the place, yet remaining steadfast. He has tireless enthusiasm for the subject matter, and to his credit he has a kind of Teflon immunity to rejection. It's hard to imagine anyone shaking off insults in such a gracious manner as he does.

It's a blessing for some, yet sad as hell, when we see Mr.

Rockoff walking around in a dazed stupor a few days after his raucous exhibition. He isn't about to get anyone's rocks off now, not even his own.

About a week into the month of June, a most unusual thing happens. I'm lying in bed, settling in for what I hope will be a night of uninterrupted sleep. Insomnia is still a bother, but it doesn't pack the same punch as before. I know I can handle it without it ruining the next day, and I don't have the disturbing nighttime thoughts anymore.

Soon I drift into sleep. But it comes to a halt when I feel the frame of the bed shake. It's like one of those vibrating beds you find in cheap roadside motels. I get up to check if the floor is shaking too, but it's not, nor is anything else in the room. I open the door and peer both ways down the hall, but there's nothing out of the ordinary. Everything is normal.

So I go back to the now still bed and search my brain for a rational explanation. I consider the possibility of an earthquake, but South Florida is far from any fault line that I know of. Besides, the shaking of an earthquake would've roused the others for sure. I wonder what else it could have been, disregarding jackhammers, tractors and locomotives, since the shaking happened in silence. There are two possibilities left. One is that I had some sort of vibratory hallucination, perhaps the product of the drugs or a sick mind. The second is that this was a gesture from the other world, maybe from God, rocking my bed in a benevolent way. To me this sounds like the best interpretation, or at least the most comforting, and it's the one I decide to go with.

I ask God to shake the bed again for proof of my theory but, sadly, it doesn't happen. Instead I'm granted a peaceful night's sleep punctuated by a dream of Lois on her 10-speed bicycle.

In the dream I'm alone, away from Danny and the car, and

I'm riding next to Lois on a bike of my own. We travel along an asphalt path through a wooded meadow. Coming up from behind, I don't recognize her at first. But then I see the side of her face with an old scar, caused by me, which now seems healed.

Seeing her again startles me with the familiar guilt and shame, but I don't look away. Our eyes meet for a moment, and I can tell she knows who I am. I half expect her to yell or scream for help, or ride off in a different direction. But she doesn't do any of that. Instead, she says something trivial, like what a nice day it is and how the path makes for a good ride. Maybe she says something more profound, but I don't remember. At the end of the conversation she says, "You can go on now."

Then I'm awake.

The dream has an intoxicating effect. To think that maybe she doesn't hate me was an altogether foreign notion until now. If dreams have any validity, then maybe in real life she doesn't hate me either. Her voice had an air of forgiveness in it, even though she didn't exactly say she forgives me. It makes me think maybe she's closer to forgiving me than I am to forgiving myself.

I think it's probably a good idea to stop crucifying myself for what I did to her. Just the thought of it, the possibility of self-forgiveness, brings me a sense of peace. The good feeling lasts throughout the day with the stride of my walking now almost spring-like.

22

J UNE 16th is the chosen date for my release from Fort
Lauderdale Hospital. The date was selected with some
degree of strategy, since my insurance coverage is running out and to stay much longer would result in my dad picking up the entire tab. This he could do for a week or so, but
beyond that the burden would be too much.

Conversations occurred between my father and Dr. Frei
about what to do from here if the insurance stops and I'm still
sick. The only viable option is a state hospital. Most likely it
would be the South Florida State Hospital in Pembroke Pines,
which is a dilapidated 350-bed facility built in 1957. As a rule,
these places do little more than serve as human storage ware-
houses with mandated drugging for all. It's easy to see how being incarcerated there would result in a downward spiral into
chronic mental illness. Such is the everyday reality of things.
But, thankfully, the Pembroke Pines option doesn't materialize, at least not for now.

Going home again is a surreal concept until the day it actually happens. Armed with the medication—Trilafon, Eskalith

and Cogentin—and my scant personal belongings, I get into my mother's Mercury with no reservations about leaving this place. For three months this has been my place of residence, and not for a single day did I feel grateful for the predicament. Living at home or anywhere other than this place became an obsession. What to do after my release is a hazy concept at best. Nearly all my energy has gone into how I'd get out of here, and once that was achieved the rest would take care of itself. One of the social workers asked me what I might do when I get home, to which I said, "I'll clean my room." Beyond that, the future is vague.

The ride home should be a joyful experience, but it isn't. I feel relieved, of course, but not much else. My mother told the staff that she's worried about me decompensating back into florid psychosis, and who could blame her given my recent track record? She also complained about my lack of a coherent plan for the months ahead. She knows that if anything goes wrong she's on the front line, and her attitude isn't much different from a soldier preparing for the next defensive maneuver. When, where and how the battle might occur are the kinds of preoccupations she must have right now.

She can take small comfort in the fact that she's been battle-tested, having earned her mettle in these types of situations. Unlike a soldier, though, my mother's strategy is to mother me the best way she knows, which is a good thing. It's what I need to rebuild my shattered confidence.

True to word, I start my new life by cleaning my old room. The last night I spent here was the night I demolished the place and, although my mother cleaned up after that, I want to rearrange things to help sever the connection with my night of violence. Just as I did in my pre-high school days, I move the furniture, this time with the bed along the opposite wall from the window and the desk facing the window.

From all the time spent in confinement, I've come to develop an appreciation for windows and what's beyond them. My bedroom window looks out upon a thick mat of St. Augustine grass and the fence and the gate where Phil broke his arm. There's also a row of bushes separating our property from the neighbors and a couple of palm trees. Ten or so feet beyond my window is a small depression in the ground where there used to be a sandbox. Next to the old sandbox was a rabbit hutch my father built when we first took residence in the house. Like the sandbox, it was dismantled and taken away a few years ago.

Similar to life in the hospital, I find sleep a compelling diversion from the boredom of life. My typical daily pattern is to get up at around eleven o'clock, make breakfast, walk around dazedly looking for something productive to do, and then by two o'clock it's back to bed for a nap. The sound of my sister Julia in the kitchen usually rouses me up. If guests are here, I get a feeling of shame for my laziness and if the shame is strong enough I get up and make an effort at social interaction. But the ability to make small talk is lost to me. More than a few minutes of it and I'm wrapped in a web of nerves.

At the hospital I didn't realize how inept I've become in conversing and handling the responsibilities of life. There, everything was structured into a simple routine, which included breakfast, recreational therapy, a meeting with Dr. Frei, lunch, group therapy, dinner and family visits. When an activity wasn't structured in, I could sleep or pace or play cards with another patient. As a last resort, I could always zone out in front of a window. That was the extent of my decision-making burden.

The place offered no incentive for independent living. In fact, it fostered dependency on the staff, and—as logic would dictate—the longer you stay, the more dependent you get. In total, I was hospitalized for nearly six months, during which time I didn't need to make a single important decision. If I had stayed another six months, the staff would need to tell me when to wipe my ass.

One day, not long after my release, my lack of will becomes painfully clear. Julia has been driving my father's old truck—a 1977 Chevy Blazer—and there's something wrong with its air conditioning system. Maybe it needs a Freon recharge or a new belt or, at worst, a compressor. As a helpful big brother, not wanting my sister to get taken in by unscrupulous mechanics, I go with her to the garage to make sure they do the right thing.

We pull up to the shop whereupon the mechanic asks me what the problem is. I speak, but the words come out weak and scattered. The more I talk the more I work myself into linguistic contortions. Realizing what a bumbling fool I seem to be, the mechanic looks away in frustration and then asks for clarification from Julia. She takes over and explains the problem with the full faculty of her reasoning. The mechanic thanks her and takes the keys.

I feel about two feet tall.

A week or so later, my maternal grandfather shows up at the house. He knows how unproductive I've been since returning home, and he aims to do something about it. He decides to teach me the art of charcoal sketching.

Together we sit at the kitchen counter with all the necessary implements in perfect order. My grandfather starts with the basics of shading and using the eraser in the proper way. Then he tells me about the different intensities of charcoal while doing a sample sketch of a tree or a woman's face, making it look easy. "It's as simple as that," he says.

I try to do likewise but fail miserably. My hand trembles and as soon as I start drawing I forget the fundamentals just demonstrated by my grandfather. The end result is an embarrassing mess. I get up without excusing myself and cool off in the swimming pool.

From the pool, I can hear my mother explaining to my

grandfather how I can't handle so much at once and how easily overwhelmed I get. It's like she's talking about a helpless
child.

In the first month out of the hospital, I get a few calls and
visits from old friends. It's foolish to go out of my way for
them after they've ignored me the past six months. I don't
want to tell them how angry I am about it, since that would
only lead to bullshit excuses I don't want to hear. So I put
on a nice face whenever we get together, which doesn't help.
Hearing all these pleasant words come out of my mouth while
ignoring the hard truth is something I'm used to, and I'm used
to the self-disgust that comes with it. It's a struggle to be so
phony.

Rather than putting myself through all that crap, I drift back
to the safety of home and family and, especially, my mother.
At the age of 19 I'm back to being a mamma's boy, and my
mother is all too willing to accommodate the role.

At an earlier time in life, I struggled to break free of the
mamma's boy role. It happened around age nine while lying
in bed. There I summoned up a newfound courage to confront
my mother. Up to that point, there was a bedtime ritual during
which she came into my room, sat at my bedside and gave me
a good night kiss. As fine as that might've been at age six or
seven, I grew tired of it by the time I was nine, and it came to
be a thing I detested more and more each night, as if the next
kiss would smother the life out of me. So on that particular
night, I decided to take preemptive action before she had a
chance to come in with the kiss. I knew if I waited for her to
come to me, I'd lose the strength to resist.

I got out of bed and found my mother sitting at the piano in
the living room, playing a classical piece. She stopped playing
when she noticed me standing there and not lying in bed, as I
should be. Then, in a sudden burst of bravery, I said, "No more

good night kisses!" After she agreed to my demand, I marched back to bed victorious. From that night forward I paved a new course for myself—onward to mature independence. That is, until now.

It's easy to slip back into the mamma's boy role. There are nights I cry and proclaim to my mother how pathetic I've become. Everything feels like a mess, and I'm too dumb with gloom to do anything about it. I let her comfort me, which she does with the full gift of her attention. She listens in a loving way, the way only a mother can. And she cries with me, which makes me realize how much she cares. At times I complain of pain across my shoulders and neck, like I'm bearing the full gravity of the world, and she makes the pain go away with a massage. If I want a certain food for dinner, she prepares it. If I want her to join me for a bike ride, she stops what she's doing and rides along with me. She's my saving grace during my first month out. All I have to do is imagine how it would be without her, and that's all the convincing I need. Going back to the mamma's boy role for a while is better than going back for another round of hospitalizations.

One activity my mother pressures me into is to join her in aerobics classes at Christ Methodist Church. She says it'll do me good to get some exercise and get out of the house for a while. She's right on both counts. Only I'm not so sure her strategy of church aerobics is the way to go. For one, I'm an awkward oaf, trying to keep the beat and match the church ladies step-for-step. The second thing is the irritating music crackling out of a cheap boom box. Bad enough are songs like *Footloose* and *Ghostbusters* and *Freeze Frame*. But, worst of all, is a song by the Weather Girls called *It's Raining Men*.

During this song, a few of the church ladies giggle nervously, like it's a sin or something to have such an image afflicting their minds. Hearing it once or twice might be okay, but the instructor plays the damn song every workout to the apparent delight of everyone but me. My strategy, as the only male in here, is to stay in the back row and keep a low profile. I try to ignore the fact that the whole thing is an assault on my senses.

Fumbling off balance, trying to keep rhythm to a song I hate, repeatedly losing my timing, I look up for guidance, only to see that I'm engulfed by a sea of cellulite-stuffed spandex, jiggling and giggling. It's a new order of hell.

23

BY late July, the listless boredom reaches an intolerable level. It's a harsh reality knowing I'm in no shape to return to Auburn in the fall. I can hardly read a magazine article, let alone keep up with the demands of a college course load. So I put the plan on hold, hoping it doesn't wither away altogether. The best thing for now is to return to the work of moving furniture for Van Arsdale's Transfer. I'm on good terms with everyone there, and they'll be happy to have me back.

Sure enough, one phone call and I'm back on the payroll. In fact the boss, Mr. Van Arsdale, says he wants me to start tomorrow, which I agree to in the flattery of the moment. I would've preferred to start next week. That way I could practice getting up earlier in the morning instead of my slovenly eleven o'clock wake-up. Now I'll have to jump right into the flow. The good part is I won't lie sleepless in bed, night after night, calculating the ways I could fail at this next venture.

At bedtime I check and re-check my alarm clock, making sure it has the proper setting to extract me from the weight of sleep. For backup, my mother knows the absolute latest I can stay in bed, and if it gets to that point she'll come in and wrestle me up. It'll be a rude awakening however it happens.

My mother is up well before me, making sure I'm out of bed on time. She takes pains to prepare me a good breakfast, gives me money if I need it for lunch or gas and sends me off with words of encouragement.

The scene at the warehouse is nearly the same as it was in years past. A few of the old guys are gone, and there are some unfamiliar faces, which is expected with the high turnover of the moving business. Tony is still here, looking as happy as a pig in slop to see me. He gives me his trademark hard slap on the back and asks how the hell I am. "Fine," I say, but I can't match his enthusiasm.

When it comes time for job assignments, Tony picks me to ride with him, which is flattering and also a little embarrassing. I hope I don't let him down.

I'm paired up with Tony and another guy named John. We do a decent size local move using one of the straight cargo trucks instead of the semi, which is reserved for long distance hauls. Seniority on his side, Tony gets the relatively cushy job of packing the truck and calling out what he needs next, while John and I retrieve the stuff from the house. We do the grunt work, while Tony figures out where things need to go and how best to put them there.

The pattern is a time-tested formula. First we bring out mattresses and box springs, standing them upright against the far wall on a blanket. Then we grab mirrors, framed pictures and headboards, wrap them up in blankets and squeeze them in between the mattresses and springs. Tony secures the sandwiched items with a rope. Next it's time for the big stuff, or the *base* as we call it, which includes dressers, refrigerators, large desks, breakfronts, tall bookshelves and the like. The goal is to fill up the empty spaces with the most substantial thing you can fit in there. The tightest fit is the best fit because it saves space for the remaining stuff and keeps the load from shifting in transit.

After the base is packed on the truck, we stack up the boxes, heavy ones first, working our way up to the ceiling with the lighter ones. Next we pack in the large but odd-shaped items, such as couches, over-stuffed chairs, patio furniture, TV stands and whatever else looks like it might fit well in a certain spot. If the family has a piano, we have to make sure we leave enough wall space in the truck to strap it in with pads and all.

The last step in the process is to fill in the open areas with the remaining light items, which we call *trinkets* and *knick-knacks*. These are the small, stackable items, which are no worse for wear if they get knocked around a bit. They include cushions, baskets, lampshades and other stuff of this sort. We're now approaching the final stretch. Just shy of the tailgate, we throw on the disassembled bed frames and bicycles and portable TV's wrapped in leftover pads. Finally, we shut the door and lift the tailgate. We're done with the loading, ready for a break. We head for lunch with a satisfying feeling of half accomplishment.

Tony shows kingly pride after packing a tight truck—better than anyone else in the business to hear him tell it. While pulling out of the driveway he says, "Man that truck's packed tighter than a virgin," and then he laughs like a lunatic.

To distinguish one kind of moving job from another, we use a time-honored taxonomy within the trade. Or at least it seems like universal language. By far the easiest job is the *quickie*, which means only a few select items have to be moved. Since we're paid by the hour, a quickie isn't the most desirable job, but it's a refreshing break from the routine of the larger moves. The second and best category is the *smooth move*, meaning it's easy to get in and out, and the family is well organized without a lot of excess clutter. On such jobs it's typical for us to get a bonus tip, maybe five or ten dollars apiece, after everything is delivered to the client's satisfaction. This puts us in high spirits on the drive back to the warehouse.

Toward the opposite end of the scale is the *shit job*, where there are a few undesirable factors involved, such as stairs, elevators, poorly packed boxes and a lot of knick-knacks, which makes loading the truck more tiring. Somewhere between the smooth move and the shit job is the standard, typical move.

At the negative extreme, fortunately rare, is a job we call the *cluster fuck*. This is akin to cleaning up after a train wreck. It's a case of disorganization degenerating into chaos, maddening in all aspects.

On one such job, the initial tour of the place featured a screaming naked baby running around the house while the TV blared. Half-packed boxes were scattered about the place with junk, mostly toys, strewn in every direction. The obese mother showed us around, pointing with her lit cigarette to items she was leaving for the next lucky occupants. Filth and stink were the order of the day, and this woman thought nothing of packing perishables into boxes that likely wouldn't be opened for weeks. To enter this family's world for the day was to lose faith in humankind.

It takes a few days for me to get back into the rhythm of the work, yet I realize I'm profoundly slower than I was in previous summers. I have to rest more often, drink more water and walk at a slower pace. At times I'm afraid of losing my balance, and I picture myself collapsing forward onto a new TV or some equally prized item. To keep that from happening, I check and re-check my steps whenever I'm carrying something of value.

More troubling than the lower quality of my work is the shift in my personality from summers past. Once spontaneous and funny, able to match wits with the other movers, I'm now struggling with the simplest of conversations. The new guys don't notice or care, probably figuring me to be a lifelong dullard. Maybe they think my highest aspiration in life is to someday rise to the stature of truck packer or driver of the big rig. When I tell John I graduated from high school and passed a term at Auburn, he looks like he's blown a head gasket.

Tony knows right away that something's different, and it isn't for the better. During my second week on the job, he approaches me and lets it out, telling me I've changed, asking me, "What the hell's wrong with you?" He says he misses the way I was before, which makes him reminisce about the good old days. Now he says, "You're too deep-shit serious. You need to lighten up." At one point he thinks maybe I'm stoned, so he checks my eyes for redness and asks if I'm stashing anything. After verifying that I'm clean, Tony says I need to get laid, no doubt about it. To him getting laid is the ultimate panacea, sure to cure whatever ails you.

I stay quiet during his inquisition, hoping it'll blow over soon. But I know Tony, and I know he won't let up. There's nothing I can say short of the truth that would satisfy him.

The next time we're alone, I tell him in rough detail what happened. Starting with Lois and her bicycle and the attorneys and then, moving from one hospital to another, I give a flat account of how I lost touch with reality, like it's the natural order of things. The story is scattered, with big gaps from one event to another, which leaves a lot more questions than answers. The result for Tony is an overwhelming mess of information — too much information — and it isn't worthwhile for him to sort it out. He returns to his advice about getting laid and leaves it at that. "You definitely need to get fucked," he says as he's walking away.

Soon Tony stops asking Mr. Van Arsdale to put me on the truck with him. No longer the golden boy, I'm just a moving grunt. The role suits me.

Moving furniture day after day and earning a regular paycheck slowly boosts my withered confidence. It makes me
think I'm doing something worthwhile. In past summers I
considered the job a mere stepping stone from one stage of
advancement to the next. The other men at the warehouse were
beneath me back then. I forgot about them the minute I drove
my sweat-drenched body off the parking lot.

But these days I see my coworkers differently. Now they've
got something to teach, not by what they say—it's what they
do that matters. It's their daily pattern of getting the job done,
then starting the whole process over again the next day. They
have their dreams of moving on to something brighter down
the road where they won't have to break their back for a dollar.
But they aren't about to give up the daily grind for a dream.
Despite their bitching left and right, they do the work that
needs doing. They have persistence, like a warrior, which is
something I'll need if I'm ever going to make anything of myself.

I realize I can go either way from here—forward or backward—and it's backward that seems the most likely course.
My fear of going back to a world of delusion, then back to
the hospital, is always present. It keeps me paralyzed inside. I
want to scream and rage at the world, but I know I can't. I want
to cry too, but that's just as risky. For support I give myself
cliché advice, like "Suck it up!" and "Keep plugging away."

24

As summer nears its end I muster the courage for another change. My father's been pushing the idea of my taking a class or two in the fall at the local community college. It seems like a demeaning proposition at first, but my job at Van Arsdale's warms me up to it. Maybe it's the fact that my coworkers do nothing to advance themselves. Looking to the future, I can see these men 20 years from now doing the same damn thing but far worse for wear, riddled with arthritis and bulging discs. To combat these afflictions, they'll become addicted to painkillers, smoke dope and drink the edge off everyday. This is the path they're on and I'm afraid of following suit.

Sitting with my father at his dining room table, we browse the fall course catalogue for Broward Community College, or BCC, which is sometimes taken to mean Broward Country Club. Neither of us is so bold as to suggest I could handle the more rigorous academic offerings in my current stupor. To take anything beyond the simplest courses would be a setup for failure. We both know this without saying anything. If they had a course on recovering from the ills of modern psychiatry, I would jump at it. But instead, I search for a balance between the brainlessly easy and the somewhat interesting.

What my dad and I jointly agree on are Art Appreciation and Racquetball. In the optimism of the moment, I think the art class will rekindle a hint of creativity, while racquetball might help reverse my peg leg coordination. These classes are held on Tuesdays and Thursdays, leaving the other three weekdays for working at Van Arsdale's. This is to be my pattern for the next three and a half months.

Meanwhile, I faithfully meet with Dr. Frei on a weekly basis out of fear for what would happen if I failed to do so. Our encounters are awkward and formal. He writes yarns on his yellow legal pad, and I sit across from him, wrapped in nerves, saying only the things I know he wants to hear. He feeds me positive sentiments, as if life is a bowl of cherries from here on out. But there's a catch. He says I have to stay on the drugs for at least a year after which he says, with characteristic vagueness, "We'll see."

I know better than to argue the matter. Debating would only call into question my mental stability. It would show that, after being treated by the best psychiatry has to offer, I still don't get it. I still lack insight into my illness. The concept of a chemical imbalance still hasn't sunk in. I hope it never does.

I'm at war with Dr. Frei, but now it takes the form of a standoff. On his side are the academic credentials and the scientific terminology and now my track record of apparent success on the drugs. On my side is the newly learned ability to be silent. Never underestimate the power of silence.

Another topic my father wants to discuss is what to do with my old El Camino. We both agree that it's a gas hog. And with only the bench seat and exposed cargo area, it's far from a practical vehicle. Someone could easily steal whatever's

stowed on the deck. At an earlier time in life the El Camino
suited me fine. After football practice I threw my dirty pads
back on the deck—no one on Earth would want to steal them.
On weekends, friends sat back there as we cruised up and
down the Strip. Those days are gone forever. So my dad and I
agree that I should get rid of the thing, and he'll help buy me
a more practical car.

After some searching we find a good deal on an '82 Toyota
Corolla. It's a blue five-speed with matching blue interior, two
doors and a trunk, and it couldn't be more different from the
El Camino. The car is practical, for sure, and without a hint of
character.

Going from the one vehicle to the other mirrors the kind
of change I've gone through myself. Previously animated with
a ferocity I could count on when called for—however misguided—I'm now reduced to an enfeebled type. Like the blue
Corolla, you'd hardly notice me if you tried.

The days at BCC offer a different kind of struggle from
the days of moving furniture. After breakfast, I get in my car
and drive west to Interstate 95 where I have to contend with
the madness of rush hour traffic while also re-learning how to
drive stick shift. I'm enrolled at the North Campus, which is
a bland cluster of sun bleached concrete buildings surrounded
by a large parking lot. From the outside it looks like a suburban shopping mall, minus the familiar store names.

Knowing I'll be spending a lot of time in my car, the first
task is to find a parking spot shaded from the relentless sun.
With a shortage of trees, the shaded spaces are a valuable com-
modity and are almost always taken. Most days I have to settle
for continuous direct sun rays.

With book and notebook in hand, I head upstairs to Art Appreciation class and sit away from the other students to avoid
small talk. The teacher is a young woman, hardly older than
me, who shows an awkward command of the course material.

She rarely veers from the text, which is a great relief because I wouldn't want to have to rely on my notes. My handwriting is akin to chicken scratch, barely legible, and it takes me longer than anyone else to write things down. In fact I'm stunned by the inadequacy of my writing. I think about how embarrassing it would be if anyone caught sight of the crude markings in front of me. Certifiable idiot would be the verdict. This is another reason to sit away from the others. To be certain of not being seen by the Note Police, I make walls with my forearms to hide the scrawl. With all this on my mind, appreciating the wonders of the visual arts is not high on my list of priorities.

By far the best moments in class are the times when the teacher has a slide presentation to show us. My gloom lifts when I arrive for class and—Blessed Creator—there's the projector all set up with a packed carousel. In the darkness I can forget about the faces around me and drift painlessly into the images on the screen.

The second best moment is when the bell rings, signaling the end of class. This is followed by two hours of lethargic boredom spent waiting for my racquetball class. At another time of life I might use the two hours as an opportunity to better myself in some way. Browsing the library collection, socializing in the cafeteria, lifting weights in the gym, writing letters—these are but a few of the countless ways to spend two free hours on a college campus. But I do none of these things. For me, the time is spent reclining alone in my Corolla, alternating between sleeping and listening to music. After the break, it's a taxing effort to extract my lazy body from the car and arrive on time for racquetball.

With little deviation, this is the pattern of my life through the fall semester at BCC. On the exterior it might not look so bad. I'm gainfully employed, attending college and causing no trouble for anyone, as far as I can tell. It's beyond anyone's expectations, given the first half of the year. In Dr. Frei's words, I've reached the goal of symptom stabilization, and he's mighty pleased about it.

For a while I agree that things are moving along well, like a light bulb getting brighter by the day. But soon I reach a plateau. I can see others shining brightly with what appears to be the full power of their being, while I'm locked into a low wattage existence. One night I ask my mother, "Is this the best I'm ever gonna be?" which is more of a plea than a question, since I know she can't answer with accuracy. I suppose I wouldn't complain if this is how I was all along, dimwitted from day one. But I could shine before and I remember what it was like to shine. Now I've lost it, and the reality of the loss goes deep. To regress this way, with full awareness of the regression, seems unmatched as far as life's frustrations go.

25

L IKE the rest of my family, Christine is concerned about me living the life of a joyless recluse and she wants to do something about it. On a Saturday night in late October, she and her boyfriend Billy plan a night out for the three of us at one of the popular clubs in town. My first reaction is to say no, but Christine gives me a guilt trip about how I need to lighten up. Her attitude is kind of like Tony's—*don't be so deep-shit serious and have fun for God's sake.* Billy is equally free-spirited. Together they're able to chisel away at my resistance.

The place is a glitzy, two story dance club called Confetti. It's about a mile from my house, which is perfect for walking home early in case things become intolerable. The last such place for me was the Hungry Hunter last January where things didn't turn out so well. I hope for a better outcome tonight.

We start by ordering Michelob's at the bar and walking around the place as an inseparable team. I don't want to be left alone for more than the time it takes to recycle the beer I'm drinking.

A good song plays over the sound system, so my sister grabs Billy and me to dance as a threesome. I pull back away from the shiny floor and watch them go at it for a couple of songs. But Christine isn't satisfied to have me standing on the sidelines like a petrified moron. So she trades in Billy and pulls me onto the floor.

I try to get into the groove by dancing with my sister, which is about as exciting as, well, dancing with my sister. After a couple of songs the DJ plays something obnoxious propelling the two of us back over to the bar area.

We stand around a cocktail table and yell small talk over the music. My eyes wander about the place, stopping to focus on the array of beautiful women mixed in the crowd. I catch myself dreaming the impossible dream of being with one of them. Any of them would do. They're close in terms of physical proximity, but they might as well be actresses on a movie screen as far as I'm concerned. The club would have to collapse in on itself before I'd be paired with one of these beauties. The farthest my courage takes me is the occasional solo walk through the club with glances here and there.

By around 11 P.M. the place fills to capacity with a line forming outside for latecomers. Christine challenges me to ask one of the women to dance.

"Not yet," I say, with plenty of excuses to back me up.

Then she says she'd be glad to intervene on my behalf by approaching one of them. But I say "no," terrified of the inevitable rejection. To humor her I promise to walk around the place and keep my eyes open for possibilities.

So that's what I do, delaying at various points to make it look like I'm giving it my best shot. Standing near the main bar by the entrance, I'm away from the watchful eyes of Christine and Billy. My plan is to stand here another five minutes or so, then we can all leave and I'll tell my sister how I tried but it just didn't work out.

It feels ridiculous standing here motionless, nursing a beer, looking like an outcast while everyone else is having a good time. I'm ready to head back to our table. But, just as I start to move, there's a tap on my shoulder. I turn around and see a dark-haired woman with her eyes fixed on mine.

"Hi, are you free to dance?" she asks.

At first I hesitate, wondering if this is real life or a mirage, like the sun bleached image of water on a straight highway. After the reality check I say, "Sure, I'll dance with you."

While dancing, she asks my name and tells me hers is Penny. She says she's here tonight with her sister and her sister's boyfriend, which makes me smile. Then I tell her what a coincidence that is because I'm with my own sister-boyfriend duo. We talk a little more while dancing, which messes up my rhythm, but I don't think Penny notices or cares. She tells me she's an architect and says a thing or two about a project she's been working on. I'm too stunned and nervous to retain most of what she says.

When the song is over, I think the natural course of action is to buy her a drink. But then I realize I don't have enough money in my wallet, which sends a shock wave of panic through my rib cage. I get a grip on the nerves and tell her I'll be back in a minute. Then I go over to Christine to borrow some money, which she has, thank the heavens above.

Back at the bar with Penny, I can see she has a nearly full drink, but I buy her another just the same. I can't think of anything else to do that would fit the moment. There's no place to sit, so we stand at the bar with her leaning against it. She tells me how tall I am and how thick my hair is, which makes me self-conscious and embarrassed all over again. I try to think of nice things to say to her, and there's plenty of material to work with. She has long, shiny hair with radiant, brown eyes and skin that looks velvety soft. Her figure isn't supermodel material, like what you'd find on the cover of *Glamour*. But it's a curvy, unmistakably feminine body—a sight for weary eyes. Her voice is soft with a quick wit, but she isn't overbearing.

I fumble around, thinking of nice things to say but everything I test out in my brain falls flat. So I keep the words to a minimum, hoping she'll fill the dead air with talk about herself. There are awkward moments of silence. But even so, Penny stays with me, and I can sense my confidence building.

Soon the talk is interrupted by the presence of Christine and Billy and, later, by Penny's sister and her sister's counterpart. They come partly out of nosey curiosity and partly to tell us that they're ready to leave. Penny drove herself here, and she offers to drop me off at home when we're ready to go. With this resolved, we say goodbye to the others.

Now it's just the two of us, with no sisters or sisters' boyfriends to provide a buffer. The club is winding down toward closing. The DJ gives the last call for alcohol. I want to keep the night going a little longer. With replenished confidence, I ask Penny if she'd like to go across the street with me for breakfast at Denny's.

"Sure," she says. "That sounds like fun."

Despite the fact that it would be quicker to walk, we drive over to the restaurant. It's after two o'clock, and the place is filled with late night revelers. Like us, they're clinging to the night's last chance for human contact. Some of them are raucous teenagers, yelling, smoking, cussing and generally making drunken slobs of themselves. Others are the more sedate and experienced variety, interested more in talk than showmanship. A few others are ruddy, leather-faced drunks.

The hostess leads us to a booth with a view of the intersection where Commercial Boulevard crosses Federal Highway. Penny makes a trip to the ladies room while I look at the menu and the cars idling at the signal. It's good to know that my brain is keeping up with the flow of events. It's amazing really.

She returns to the booth, and soon our coffee arrives. The

waitress sees that we're ready to place our order. Penny selects a simple omelet, while I order the French toast with sausage links.

When our food arrives, I see that hers doesn't look as appetizing as mine, so I offer her a slice of French toast. She doesn't want any, but instead of just saying no thanks, like you'd expect, she says, "Thanks, but I've already had my bread quota for the day."

The comment catches me off guard, making me laugh a little. God knows how long it's been since I've had a moment like this. Sometimes it's the simplest things. We proceed to make a running joke out of the bread quota and other such dietary restrictions. I ask if she's surpassed her heroin quota for the day, which gets her laughing pretty good.

After the meal Penny drives me home. As we approach the driveway, I tell her I'm having such a good time that I don't want her to go. Feeling the momentum on my side, I ask if she'd go with me for a walk around the neighborhood.

"I'd like that," she says.

So we walk together. The universe has definitely shifted for the better.

As we pass by Phil's house, I tell her about my friendship with him going back to age five and about some of the times we had growing up. I mention other landmarks as well, like the mighty sea grape tree we convened in after school and the house we thought was haunted on Halloween night. I tell her about Van Arsdale's too, and I say something vague about the rough times that got me off track.

She asks what my plans are for the future, and I tell her that my goal is to go back to Auburn. It surprises me how quickly I come out with the wish, but tonight it seems like a real possibility.

We walk back to her car without saying much of anything—just walking and now holding hands. Maybe we've exhausted our conversational quota for the night, or maybe it's something I said that put her in a place of silence. When we get to her car, she leans against the door without opening it.

I thank her for asking me to dance. I don't think I can thank her enough.

When she reaches for the door handle, I ask if I could kiss her. Penny doesn't say anything—she just leans her head forward and kisses me.

It's not a long kiss or one of those passionate sex kisses you see on daytime soaps, but it's the sweetest thing to come my way. Before the kiss I wasn't sure what I was—maybe half beast, half lunatic—certainly not a desirable creature. But the kiss does something to me, almost like mouth-to-mouth resuscitation, bringing a dead man back to life.

I'm buzzing with excitement, but all I can do is wave goodbye as she drives off. In my left hand is a piece of paper with her phone number, which I grip like a lifeline.

Two days after the magical night with Penny, I get up the nerve to call her. I wonder if she was only humoring me when she gave me her number, and maybe she has a boyfriend she forgot to mention. I also wonder how the hell I'll match up with the magic of our first encounter. Everything was so fluid and fresh. Finally, I tell my fear creating brain to shut up while I dial the number.

With voice quivering, I ask if she remembers me. She says of course she does and that she's glad I called. After some awkward small talk, we make plans to double date with her sister and the boyfriend serving as quasi-chaperones. Even on the phone I can sense the magic is still here. The thought of it makes my voice more confident. I think maybe she wants to see me as much as I want to see her.

The following weekend we go out as planned, and with that date's success we make arrangements for another date without the sibling accompaniment. By the third date, I can feel the relationship moving in a serious direction. I like everything about Penny, and for whatever reason she seems to like me too. It feels so different and good being around her.

But there's also a bad feeling lurking below the surface. It's the sense of being a fake, like I'm posing as a normal guy while hiding the fact of where I've been and what I've been like over the past year. There's a faraway distance I feel with Penny whenever it crosses my mind, and it's getting worse. By the fourth date I resolve to tell her the whole story and try to accept the outcome, whatever it is.

Beginning with Lois and her 10-speed bicycle, through my discharge from Fort Lauderdale Hospital and covering the drugs I now have to keep taking, I stay true to the story. At times my voice shakes, and my eyes rarely leave the carpeted floor of Penny's living room. But the story comes out a lot more smoothly than the account I gave Tony at Van Arsdale's. And, unlike Tony, Penny listens without interrupting or rushing ahead with cliché solutions. She just sits across from me and lets it sink in.

When I finish, I don't have the nerve to look her in the eyes, but I sense her looking at mine. My body is as rigid as plywood from telling the story, and I'm thinking about leaving after saying such stuff. I back up in the chair to let her know she doesn't have to give me a sympathy hug or anything like that. I've had enough patronizing gestures for a lifetime. Just to be heard is the point of it. That's enough for now.

Penny puts her head down low, breaking my gaze at the carpet. I can't help but meet her eyes with mine. "Hey there," she says to break the ice.

I say "Hey" back, so she'll know I'm still breathing.

Then she pats the cushion next to her and tells me to come over to the couch where she's sitting.

This I do gladly, but I'm still afflicted with the plywood

posture.

Once I'm seated on the couch, she holds the closer of my arms and nestles her head between my neck and shoulder. In silence, she works her hands into my fingers and slowly rocks side to side.

Everything about her is soft and warm. Her abundant hair sweeps the side of my face as we rock, and it smells sweet. We sit in silence, looking at our intertwined hands. Then I hear Penny's nose making that stuffed-up noise that comes from holding back tears, and I can see a track on her face where a tear went down. That's when I know. I really know she heard me.

With Penny's arrival the colorful aspect of life returns. Others notice the change as well. My family looks more at ease and less inclined to ask loaded questions about my state of mind. Phil and other friends call and joke around, almost as though things are back to normal. Dr. Frei shows cautious satisfaction by lowering the drugs to a more tolerable level. Moving jobs at Van Arsdale's flow more smoothly and my classes at BCC seem less oppressive, although the atrocious handwriting remains.

One night Penny invites me up to the loft bedroom of her compact apartment where she promises to give me a back rub. This is in addition to the shirt she already gave me for my 20th birthday. It's almost Thanksgiving, and soon I'll have something to be immensely thankful for.

I follow her up the ladder-type stairs and sit with her at the foot of the bed. We talk about the proper method of giving and receiving a back rub, agreeing that too much clothing would only be a hindrance.

She takes off her shoes, while I fumble like a klutz with mine. By the time I finally get my shoes off, she's already taken off her blouse, and now she's adjusting her bra. I sit still with all my energies focused on the vision of this sweet woman. Maybe I'm making her nervous because she's fiddling with her bra and it isn't going anywhere. She says it's part of a new set of lingerie she bought for the occasion and, while pretty, it isn't exactly user-friendly. I agree that it's very pretty indeed. Regarding the matter of its removal, I tell her I'm here to help. God knows that's the truth.

I find the clasps connecting the bra and work them apart. I try to show some finesse and not rush things too much, but I'm as eager as a guy can be. It feels like every cell in my body is a hormone on a mission. Together we work the straps down her arms.

The rest of the night is the finest bliss I've known. Whether or not I get the promised back rub escapes my memory. What I do remember is the boundless energy I have long after our first loving encounter. We talk into the small hours, mindless of the time, covering topics large and small. It occurs to me that Tony may have been right after all.

In my excitement, the natural thing is to talk about going back to Auburn, as if it's a quest to get back to the enchanted land of *Brigadoon*. I share my abbreviated college memories, while she shares a few of her completed memories of life at the University of Florida. She's 27, well beyond the college scene, but having been through it—and much improved as a result of it—she can appreciate my quest. Still it makes her sad. In just over a month we'll be saying goodbye.

26

B EFORE I can get too excited about my return to Auburn, I have final exams at BCC to contend with. The Racquetball exam is laughable, with the teacher casually asking us questions and rating our physical grasp of the game. But the Art Appreciation exam catches me off guard. The test is a collection of short essay questions covering the whole semester's worth of material. While other students write feverishly and complete the test in the time allotted, I struggle with every question, finding it hard to string together the simplest ideas. My clumsy handwriting haunts me throughout, and I'm afraid the teacher won't be able to read any of this gibberish. Time is racing away while I labor over my words. It's one dull word after another in a slow, painful progression. When the bell rings, I'm just over halfway done and nearly dripping with sweat from the effort.

I get up and ask the teacher if I can talk with her privately. She agrees and walks me to a corner. I tell her about my current situation and about the hard times just passed, explaining that she can even call my psychiatrist for proof. I tell her I liked the class very much and haven't missed a day of it. I finish by asking if she could please be mindful of these favorable facts when grading me, as opposed to the mangled crap I'm turning in today.

After my humiliating plea, the teacher gives me a woeful look and tells me not to worry. But worry is what I do, not so much about the class grade but about the prospect of repeating this shameful episode at Auburn.

A couple of weeks after finals I get the envelope with my grades. I receive B's for both classes, which gives me a sense of relief. But in the back of my mind, I know that to be successful down the road I'll need access to the full capacity of my brain. Toward that end, a risk will be necessary. Someday soon I'll have to risk dumping the medication.

Early in January 1985, Phil and I load our respective cars and head north in the direction of Auburn just as we did this time last year. The goodbyes and well wishes are over; it's time to move on. The hardest goodbye occurred yesterday when I met with Penny over lunch. I wanted to keep it short because I was afraid that if I stayed too long I'd never want to leave. I promised her I'd keep in touch and, after a clumsy pause, I kissed her lips for the last time. She was unusually quiet. She knew there wasn't any stopping me, so why drag it out?

The sadness of her face stayed with me throughout the night, and I could barely sleep. Now I've got a 650-mile trek in front of me and a terrible longing in my heart. I hope the drive will help ease the pain.

For Phil this is a routine trip, but he knows the importance it holds for me. With his radar detector on high, Phil leads the way, stopping for gas and then for supper in Tifton, Georgia. There we find Shoney's restaurant, just off the interstate, and we both order the all-you-can-eat buffet, where we also have our fill of all-you-can-drink sweet tea.

Famished from the long journey, we eat like pigs in hog heaven, and when we're both thoroughly satiated we call up familiar Southern expressions to fit the moment. "I'm 'onna bust a gut," I say, with the words strung together in a low redneck drawl, belly jutting out.

We rehearse the line until we get it just right, and we practice a few other Southernisms for good measure. The waitress probably thinks we're retarded, but I don't care. For me it's a rite of passage. It's like knowing the password for entry into another land.

My new living quarters are back at CDV in a different apartment with a new set of housing mates. By this time Phil lives in a posh, off-campus condominium on a lake—thus the path of upward mobility never failing him. My new roommate is a mechanical engineering student who has all the personality of a mechanical engineering student. We probably say a total of 15 words to each other the whole academic term.

I get along better with one of the suitemates in the adjacent bedroom. He's a tall, lanky guy named Rick with a Howdie Doodie face, minus the freckles. Rick is nice to everyone, as far as I can tell. He's the kind of guy who doesn't have enemies.

Other than his friendly disposition, the most notable thing about Rick is the fact that he eats fried bologna. Maybe it's a delicacy in his hometown or, more likely, maybe it's the best that'll do in a pinch. His method is to heat up a Teflon-coated frying pan and put the slice of bologna in it with a cut along a radius line, so it won't curl up and make a bologna bowl. Instead, the radial cut recedes into a V, making the bologna look like a brown Pac Man. Once a certain smell is achieved, Rick flips the slice over until the other side's cooked too. Throw on a slice of cheese, put it between two slices of Wonder Bread, and it passes for a meal.

On the academic front I sign up for a full load of courses, which consists of English Composition, World History, Introductory Sociology and another sociology course with a different guest speaker every week. One might say I have a slight edge in two of these classes because they're repeats from last winter. But given my state of mind then *and* now, this isn't much of an advantage.

Another thing I do is return to the ATO fraternity, where I agree to go through their initiation ritual if they'll have me back. During one of their chapter meetings, with Phil rallying my support, the brothers voted me back in. I'm not sure if Greg the pencil-neck prick was there at the meeting—probably not, given my favorable outcome. It's good to hear that Deano pledged the fraternity as well. With five other pledges, Deano and I are slated to go through initiation later in the quarter.

The first bad thing to happen comes as no big surprise. It's the painful realization that I can't keep pace with the history professor. The class is held in a large auditorium with 200 or more students, all writing in a frenzy to match the teacher's manic style. Just like at BCC, my notes are abysmal. As I project into the future, I can't fathom getting away with the kind of stunt I pulled in the Art Appreciation class. This professor doesn't appear to be the merciful type, and I doubt he'd show much favor to a downtrodden freshman on neuroleptic drugs. He'd probably say something demeaning like, "If you don't think you can handle the work here, maybe you should try a community college." Hearing words like that would cut me to the bone. The best thing for now is to avoid him altogether and withdraw from his class, which is what I decide to do.

On the same day, I make another key decision—one that goes counter to the advice of the medical establishment. Despite the ominous warnings of Dr. Frei, I decide to stop taking the drugs. He warned me about the temptation of doing this, citing the high statistical likelihood of a trip back to the psychiatric ward. I don't doubt his statistics and up to now his warnings have assured my total compliance. But with time and distance separating us, Dr. Frei's words are less threatening. From where I stand, the advantages of drug free living outweigh the fear induced warnings of psychiatry. I'll take the risk, and no one else will know about it.

The conservative and intelligent course of action would be to taper off the drugs slowly over a period of a few weeks. That's the medically advisable thing to do whenever drugs such as these are stopped. But my temperament isn't geared for such a strategy, especially after the day's humiliation. Instead, I decide to flush everything down the toilet.

With the apartment free of roommates, I gather up the bottles and enter the bathroom, locking the door behind me. One by one, I pour out the contents of the three bottles—Trilafon, Eskalith and Cogentin—taking notice of the various shapes and colors, especially the bright yellow and gray. For effect, I let the capsules sit awhile so the gelatin has a chance to expand and distort. The inside of the toilet looks like an Andy Warhol pop art display. Despite my feeble grasp of art appreciation, it's a scene I can appreciate. Then there's the flush—and a whirl of color—which is ironic because the drugs did anything but provide a whirl of color while I was taking them. It's good riddance at last.

To play it safe, I keep the empty bottles hidden in a locked toolbox in case I need to get refills. To exercise that option is almost unthinkable.

After the pills are gone and the bottles locked away, I wonder whether this was such a good idea after all. I wish I could tell someone about it. I wish Penny were here. I could tell her what I've done without fear of her calling Dr. Frei and ratting me out. She's probably the only one I could tell.

I sit on my bed, lonely, wondering what's in store for me.

Have I just made the biggest mistake of my life? I don't know if I could take another round of psychosis. But even more than that, I'm afraid of the oppression of the mental ward and a return to the same mind-stripping drugs. And the thought of seeing Dr. Frei again, visiting me in the seclusion room, is the scariest predicament of all. Hearing his contorted language about getting me stabilized again would just about kill me.

To get the upper hand on my fear, I go for a walk. If there's anything in this life I've learned, it's the value of walking. I want to walk the entire campus. I want to announce to the world that I'm here, at Auburn University, and not in a god-damn mental ward. No fucking shrink is gonna take me away from this place. This is where I belong!

The walk takes me through the majority of campus, and it's invigorating. With each step, I feel like I'm claiming this as my territory. I walk until my feet are sore and my eyes tired. Now I can go back to the apartment and sleep without such a heavy burden.

The very next day I get a letter from Penny. In it she says she wishes things could be different and that the two of us could've stayed together in Fort Lauderdale, but she understands what I have to do for myself, and it makes her sad to know she's not a part of it. She ends the letter by saying she doesn't want to get her hopes up and so insists that I not write or call her back.

I read the letter over a few times, then lock it away in my toolbox with the empty bottles. It feels cruel not to write her back, and yet what is there to say? I think maybe I love her, but I also think the love would turn sour if I sacrificed my plans for her. Maybe it's best to keep quiet and not acknowledge the love at all. Or maybe it's just easier that way. I'll remember the good times we had, and in time the pain will ease. This is what I tell myself.

But I think about Penny a lot, and I miss her. She guided me out of a dark time, which may not be over. I feel like I still need her support, especially now that I've flushed the drugs. But she can't help anymore. From here, I need to go it alone. There's no Penny to support my heart and no drugs to quell my brain.

Nothing remarkable happens the day after I dump the drugs, and nothing bad happens during the days and weeks after that. Slowly, my energy level and my handwriting return to normal. But the big stuff, the psychotic stuff, doesn't return...at least not for now.

It's a strange phenomenon, walking around campus, going to class, talking to friends, partying on the weekends and going to basketball games while simultaneously wondering and worrying whether or not I'll go psycho at some point. It's always in the back of my mind, and the thought of it happening again puts a strange spin on life. I carry around a kind of curse that no one else knows about. Some of the students know about the craziness last year, but no one knows that I flushed the drugs. And, understandably, no one asks about this curse of probabilities—the weight of wondering day after day whether it'll happen again. Statistics are a part of my new life. What is the statistical probability that I'll make a return to the nuthouse?

The voice of reason says that the longer I go without such an episode, the less likely it is to happen again. So with each day that it doesn't happen, the curse recedes, little by little. That's what I tell myself. It's a private battle against the curse. No one can fight it but me. The necessary tools are time and the fighting spirit. But fear is a part of it too. The fear and the curse are always there, lurking in the background.

27

ABOUT a month after returning to Auburn, I get a phone call from my attorney regarding the civil suit Lois filed against Danny and me. He says the matter was handled out of court with a final settlement to be paid at once. The settlement amount is only a curiosity for me now because it'll be paid by the insurance company and not by my father. I want to know the amount but don't ask, and the lawyer doesn't volunteer the information.

Later, Danny would tell me that the figure is in the ballpark of $900,000. I'm sure a good chunk of it goes to the attorneys. Another sizable chunk is probably earmarked for Lois' medical expenses, although I never get these details.

With the case finally over, I hope Lois is able to gain some satisfaction. And with the boost of income she can probably make a better life for herself. Not knowing the facts, this is how I imagine it to be.

The old feelings of shame and guilt connected with the incident are mostly gone now. But if I think about it long enough, they come back to the surface. Like a scar they're never really gone, and that's probably how it should be.

Midway through the winter term, Deano and I prepare for the fraternity's initiation. We've heard rumors of how treacherous the ordeal can be and how some of the pledges fail to make it through. Or rather, we heard about frightened pledges turning their asses and running in fear of what might happen to them. Mostly these are just scare tactics.

The two legitimate pieces of information are that, throughout initiation, we'll have to wear formal attire to classes and we won't get much opportunity for sleep. Both notions irritate me because I hate dressing up, and I don't function well without sleep.

There's a hard-edged aspect to the initiation, but it's nothing compared to being hospitalized, medicated and restrained against your will. By comparison, this is a cakewalk. We spend most of our waking hours memorizing idealistic passages written by the founding fathers and cleaning the fraternity house inside and out. We're not allowed to take showers, and we have to set up camp and take care of business in the women's bathroom, which turns into a place of refuge from the hovering brothers. To combat our mounting odor, we take French baths at the sink and we spray all sorts of masking scents into the air. The smell of concentrated evergreen will forever be imbedded in my brain as an ATO initiation odor.

There are group activities with the brothers that I won't mention, but none of these rise to the level of hazing, at least not to me. As promised, we have to don our formal attire to class. It's a way of announcing our rising stature to the lay community, and it makes us feel separate from the rest of the student body. Skipping classes for any reason is not permitted.

I find out the hard way that hitchhiking to class isn't permitted either. Yet hitching a ride becomes a must because the goddamn dress shoes I'm wearing give me blisters. It's as if there are steel spikes sewn into the leather, poking at my nerves with every footfall.

After hitching to class and back, one of the brothers sees me getting out of a car. He looks at me but doesn't say anything. In our evening meeting the truth of my transgression comes out, and the brothers turn it into an opportunity for public ridicule. I take the ridicule with pride, knowing I'll hitchhike again tomorrow if given the chance. Fortunately, Band-Aids come to my rescue.

Deano and I complete the initiation feeling proud but also hungry, smelling of foulness and drop-dead tired. Back at CDV, we order and eat the largest Domino's pizza we can get, then collapse for what must be 10 or 12 hours of undisturbed sleep. My dreams are full of Greek symbolism and platitudes from the founding fathers.

But in a matter of weeks, the creed and all the other quotes I hammered into my brain are gone from memory. For some reason, though, I'm still able to recite the Greek alphabet.

In the fall of '85 I live in the fraternity house, which proves to be academically unwise. There's a party somewhere in the house nearly every night, and there's this cute sorority girl who knocks on my door whenever she feels like it, which is often. She doesn't care about waking me out of a sound sleep because she knows her seductive power. I tell her to go away, that I need my sleep, but she keeps knocking. To stop the knocking, I let her enter my tiny room so I can tell her face-to-face how important it is that I sleep.

But this girl doesn't listen very well. Usually, in a matter of no more than a minute, she's sitting on my lap, showing me her ample cleavage. And then that's the end of my self-control. Sleep can wait.

I resort to napping during the day and not studying, as I

should be. When I do study, it's hard to ignore the chatter up and down the hall. Looking out the window, I can see guys tossing a football, running pass patterns, and I wonder how they ever get their work done. These are the same guys who brag about how long it'll take them to get their bachelor's degrees—five, six, seven years and counting. Maybe their goal is to hide out here at the frat house for as long as humanly possible. Meanwhile, I feel like a nerd for even posing as a serious student.

By the end of the term I'm tired of the whole organization. Despite the high aspirations of the fraternity's founding fathers—all of whom are long dead—the best I can manage here is sleep-deprived mediocrity. I feel like I'm forfeiting my own truth just to go along with the group. In this regard, it feels like the mental hospital all over again. Of course, I can't confess these thoughts to the brothers. I take the coward's way out and disappear without explanation. I pack my things and walk out the back door, never to return.

For the rest of my Auburn experience, I'll be living solo in a low rent trailer off Wire Road with a black cat named Rhonda. Except for classes, sporting events and occasional parties, I avoid group activities and keep my friendships to a minimum, knowing how quickly they can turn when things get rough. I become a loner—me and my cat. And it's the best way for now.

Soon my academic focus and grades improve. I begin working part-time for an entomology professor in his greenhouse where I grow collard plants and harvest cocoons for a research project he's working on. I know nothing about the project, other than the fact that it requires a bunch of collard plants and harvested cocoons.

The professor is a strange old man who takes pride in his assortment of moths, some of which are huge by moth standards. One day he demonstrates how to squeeze a certain type of moth in just the right way, so its insides jut out to make a big ball of puff. It's impressive how he does this, and he wants me to give it a try, but I decline. I figure it isn't the sort of skill I'll put to use in my spare time.

As a sophomore I realize criminology isn't the path for me. For one thing I'm not afraid of going to jail anymore, which may be why I've lost interest in the field. Second, I can't think of a decent job one might get with a degree in criminology. There's nothing here that inspires me anymore. A change is definitely warranted.

Choosing an academic path is difficult. With all the available majors, it's hard committing to just one. It's like going to the food court in a mall where there are 10 vendors, all of which seem equally appealing or unappealing, depending on your point of view. The problem is the vast array of options and the weight of indecision.

Back in high school I used to draw fairly well, and I had built things from otherwise wasted materials found around the house. With this in mind, I think industrial design might be the best choice. And it's a good choice for a while. It forces me to take courses I'd otherwise try to avoid, like trigonometry, calculus and physics, in addition to the core design and drafting classes. It also leads to the fun experience of my dad and me building a drafting table in his garage.

The creative part of designing never-before-seen objects is exciting, bringing forth skills I never knew I had. But the tedium of drafting ultimately pushes me out of the field. Near the middle of my junior year I make another change for the last time.

When I finally settle on psychology, it seems like the inevitable thing to do, like a force you resist with full knowledge that it'll get you in the end. The choice has a lot to do with my curse. I figure if I can convince the professors of a psychology department that I'm mentally stable, then maybe I can convince myself too. But it's more than that. I want to know what *really* happened to me when I went crazy, and I want to prevent it from ever happening again. That'll be my revenge. I could also say that I want to be a psychologist because, having been there, I can better identify with patients' problems, but that motive doesn't really occur to me, at least not for now. Revenge and redemption are the primary goals.

Psychology has a reputation as a cushy major here at Auburn, which is better known for its rigorous schools of engineering, architecture and veterinary medicine. The liberal arts are seen by many as a kind of dreamy cop-out, mostly chosen by female students who want to marry engineers. This bias is in the back of my mind too, and I need to get past it.

Soon I realize that a bachelor's degree in the field is little better than worthless. To really make it in this profession, I'll have to go on to graduate school after Auburn. To accomplish that, I'll need to improve my grades and do some ass kissing in the psychology department.

With renewed focus, I develop the habit of getting straight A's, quarter after quarter. I also get into the enjoyable habit of playing racquetball with one of my professors even though he wins nearly every game, and I'm not trying to lose on purpose. I do some volunteer work as well, and I join the school's psychology club, which serves no apparent function other than to enable you to say that you're a member of the club.

28

TIME can be measured in any number of ways. Although the calendar on the wall says it's June 1986,
I often use my own system of reckoning with time.
One method is to figure out how long it's been since my breakdown. A second is to discern the time passed since I flushed
my drugs down the toilet, which is now nearly 18 months and
counting. More important than the passage of time is the fact
that, despite Dr. Frei's warnings, I haven't gone psycho.

I consider this comforting thought as Deano knocks on the
flimsy door of my trailer. His visit is a nice interruption from
my solitude and better than usual because the two of us have a
week off between spring and summer quarter with no immediate plans. We sit for a while, drinking Budweisers, listening to
music and discussing how songs have changed from the 70's
to the 80's. This leads to the subject of Deano growing up in
a town where there was nothing to do but spend hours upon
hours listening to records with his brother. "Jesus, that could
get old," I say, thinking of this as an unacceptable way for me
to spend a break from classes. Then a kind of outlandish idea

occurs to me. "Hey," I say, "let's get the hell out of here and drive up to New York City."

"What, are you nuts?" he says.

"Maybe, but you gotta admit it's better than sitting around here with nothing to do. And when have you ever been to New York?"

"Never" is his response, which paves the way for decisive action. Within two hours, we're packed and on the road under starlight, heading north on Interstate 85. Once we're beyond Washington, DC, every subsequent mile marks a northernmost frontier for Deano. Bleary-eyed and exhausted, we get as far as Princeton, New Jersey before settling for the cheapest dirt-bag motel we can find on the outskirts of town.

Next morning we awaken with exciting plans for the city. It feels like this huge mega-magnet is drawing us in. There's no turning back. With my blue Corolla we snake through the Holland Tunnel into Lower Manhattan, emerging into a buzz of sensory overload. The first thing is the traffic, which to me isn't a big deal. Negotiating a specific route is not a priority. The key thing is we're here. I explain to Deano that as long as we manage to stay on the Island we can't be lost. The issue of parking however is a big deal, especially with our skimpy budget and complete lack of city sense. If we were more savvy tourists we would've dropped the car off in Newark and taken the train in, but fresh from Alabama that's asking a bit much.

We luck into a spot in Chelsea, near the youth hostel where we're supposed to sleep for the night. For the price of $14 per person with college ID, we get a bunk and access to a community bathroom and a tiny kitchen. With these essentials covered, we set out on foot to explore the city. I resent the fact that I'm carrying my clunky Nikon camera around my neck, looking so much the part of a tourist, but I resolve to take enough shots to make it worthwhile. I capture the sights at Washington Square and along the streets of SoHo. In Chinatown Deano gets a craving for egg-rolls, which taste delicious mostly because they're from Chinatown. On the way to Battery Park, we stop at the World Trade Center to marvel at the amazing height of the twin towers. Standing almost precisely between them, I snap a picture of the parallel lines shooting skyward in convergence but stopping just short of the scant clouds. The effect is almost mesmerizing. I had been here once before with my aunt and cousin intent on dining at the Windows on the World restaurant, but the maitre d' refused us since I was wearing jeans and in clear violation of the dress code. That made me feel like shit. Today, however, the issue is money and the fact that we have very little of it.

The next stop is Battery Park, where we take photos in front of the Statue of Liberty before boarding a subway uptown toward Rockefeller Center. Walking up Fifth Avenue instills in me a powerful feeling that's hard to shake. It's a sense of being in a low class, much closer to poverty than I've ever felt before, and a big zero in the eyes of my fellow pedestrians. Among the glitzy storefronts, where everything is beyond my price range, I'm ashamed of how little I actually have. This street is beautiful and dazzling and humiliating all at the same time.

After a cheap meal, courtesy of street vendors, Deano and I wash up at the hostel in preparation for a night on the town. A pretty cashier at a record store suggests a place called Danceteria on 30th Street, which isn't a bad walk from here. As we stroll up Eighth Avenue, we speak with a kind of super charged intensity filled with the fresh panorama of the city. Deano calls the place a "nonstop caffeine buzz." I say that's as good a description as any.

The club is a three story behemoth, loud enough to peel paint, with something different on each floor, but I never make it beyond floor number one. The first task is to acquire a couple of beers for Deano and me, which is not an easy thing. As the more aggressive of the two, it's my job to push and compress myself forward to the bar among a throng of thirsty patrons. Then there's the issue of price—five dollars for a Budweiser, which is nearly five times what I'd have to pay in Auburn. It looks like we won't be getting drunk tonight.

Nursing our beers, Deano and I head toward the stairwell to survey the entire club. In my peripheral vision I catch two attractive women looking over at me from the bar, and they seem to be talking about me. It would be foolish not to say anything. I push my way closer and say, "Hi, where you from?"

One says she lives near Tompkins Square, and the other says something I can't make out. Revealing that I drove up from Alabama seems to raise my stock in their eyes, but the same information coming from Deano doesn't impress. In fact they seem repulsed by him, which could certainly hurt my chances. When the shorter of the two asks if I'd like to go with them to another club without Deano, I realize a quick decision must be made. I know it's impulsive and mean, but I agree to ditch Deano in favor of these two beauties. I tell him I'll be back by midnight.

The place they take me to is a semi-private club overlooking Times Square. It's up on the 17th floor of a building shaped to match the angle of Broadway intersecting Seventh Avenue. I think the place is called Nirvana or, if not, that's what it should be called. Decorated with Asian flare and a warm red hue, it's a stunning contrast from the Danceteria. The two most notable features are the dance floor and the dimly lit room designated as the place to smoke marijuana or anything else a person might want to smoke. It's also the place for couples to make out.

After a trip to the men's room, I find myself sitting in the pot smoking room, wondering where the girls went, but not really caring as the wafts of smoke penetrate my brain. Someone I don't recognize hands me a cold Heineken, which I accept with deepest gratitude. Another person offers me a hit off his joint. I decline, saying "not necessary."

Time seems to move at a different pace here. I get it in my head that there's no rush and no need to fuss. That sounds about right—no rush, no fuss—my new mantra. Concern over Deano completely escapes my mind.

I move slowly toward the multi-windowed dance floor and am captivated by the bustling streets below. Thoughts of Fifth Avenue return as I gaze down at the people strolling on the sidewalks. Standing here in this den of opulence and excess, I don't feel so estranged from the source of it all, whatever that might be.

"Hey, you know anybody down there?" says a woman sitting just a few feet behind me. I can tell by her tone that she's sort of teasing me, and I like it.

"Not likely," I say, giving up on a witty response.

She asks if I'm enjoying my Heineken. To which I answer, "Of course." It then dawns on me that she had the beer delivered to me by a friend of hers who happens to be sitting across from her. "Wow, thank you," I say, "I figured maybe it was free Heineken night, but apparently not."

The woman introduces herself as Carolyn and then tells me the names and various occupations of the people around us. While pretending to listen, I'm also pondering the whereabouts of the two women who brought me here. For whatever reason they've apparently ditched me. But this Carolyn, though older and less attractive, seems pretty interested. When she asks if I would be willing to join her and some friends for a trip to one of her favorite nightclubs, I give her an excited "yes."

At street level, we board multiple cabs headed for a place called the Red Parrot on West 57th Street. Carolyn is crammed in between me and another guy whose name I'm supposed to know. We arrive at the bar at around 1:30 A.M. and the place is still packed. The well tailored bouncer apparently knows Carolyn, and he nods us all in with a smile. Once inside, I find myself captivated by the hugeness of the place, and yet it all fits together into a flashy, zap-your-brain kind of elegance. An enchanted use of light plays off the reflective walls, one of which has projections of the city skyline. Two massive cages with live parrots border the parquet dance floor, and there's a stage featuring its very own big band orchestra. This place is amazing.

Better yet are the people, especially the women, dressed like runway models under a moving spotlight. Carolyn notices my head shifting from one female ideal to another, and she asks if this club is anything like I'd find in Alabama. The question is absurd, but its intent is to get me focused back on her, and I comply.

I can't quite decide if Carolyn is attractive. Certainly, it's unfair to compare her to some of these women, all of whom must've been hand selected by the doorman for their statuesque beauty. But she does have a kind of sexy appeal. Her long black hair, her sensuous eyes and her thick red lips adorn a body that is slender and fit. She's probably in her late 30's, far too old for me, but we're only talking about tonight. After a few more drinks and dances and loud conversation, Carolyn announces to the group that she's ready to go home. And she wouldn't mind a ride from me.

We taxi over to my car in Chelsea and drive up along the Henry Hudson Parkway to the George Washington Bridge, crossing over the Hudson into Fort Lee, New Jersey, where we park on the street next to Carolyn's apartment. She invites me in and proceeds to kiss me in her living room while unbuckling my belt. I'm amazed at how much energy I still have, and I'm now convinced that she is indeed attractive. We amble over to her plush, king bed and nestle in for some moments of sexual passion. Then I drift off for what can't be more than three hours of sleep.

I awaken to the aroma of coffee and to the sight of Carolyn in a sleek robe, walking toward me with a book. It bears the title *She's Okay, Let Her In*, with the subtitle *The Inside Story on the Night People*. And there on the back cover is a chic photo of Carolyn, posing with a mink shawl. "Wow, this is you!" I say, stating the obvious.

Then she tells me about the research that went into the book's creation. The strangeness of it all starts sinking in. Two days ago I was alone in my trailer, relaxing after final exams. Now I'm lying in the bed of New York City's self-proclaimed queen of the nightclub scene. What a strange and amazing shift. Carolyn continues her story. I think she senses that I'm listening with real interest, which prompts her to give me a complimentary copy. I thank her accordingly.

With a new sense of urgency about getting back to Deano at the hostel, I shower, get dressed and eat a nicely prepared breakfast as fast as I can without looking too rushed. After a series of goodbye kisses, I'm back on the road, driving at over 70 miles an hour down the Parkway with the photographed face of Carolyn looking up at me from the passenger seat. Quite a memorable souvenir, I'm thinking while still buzzing with excitement.

Entering the puny kitchen of the hostel, I see Deano and a few other people huddled around the toaster. It appears that toast is the sole form of sustenance here. When someone asks if I want any, my response harkens me back to Penny. "No thanks," I say, "I've already had my bread quota for the day." This time, though, there's no laughter. Nothing about it is funny.

Deano doesn't say a word. It's clear that he's pissed off. He's extremely angry with me, for one, but he's also pissed over the fact that he barely slept all night in his squeaky bunk next to a fat German who snored the entire night.

"Jesus Deano, I'm sorry," I say, but I can't help smiling a little bit as the words come out. My apology is a big fake and he knows it.

"Shut your fucking trap," he says. "Let's get out of this place."

We pack our stuff into the trunk of my car and drive uptown to Central Park West, where we find another lucky spot. It occurs to me that mine must be the only automobile in the city with Alabama plates.

We've negotiated a plan for the day, which is to walk around Midtown, do a little souvenir shopping and visit the Hayden Planetarium. The latter turns out to be a great place for both of us to catch up on much needed sleep.

Returning to the car, I'm seized by a horrible sight. The backseat passenger window has been busted open, glass strewn about the seat, with a mess of clothes spread throughout the interior. "Fuck!" I yell, loud enough for anyone with ears to hear, "Son of a fucking bitch!"

Further investigation reveals that the stolen items include my collection of cassette tapes, Deano's clothes, the Rockford Fosgate amplifier, which had been mounted under my seat, and my Nikon camera, equipped with all the fabulous photos I shot yesterday. That's the hardest one to swallow—my beautiful memories annihilated by one terrible act. It feels like a violation, like a rape. If I had the power to negotiate with the fucker (or fuckers) who did this I would ask, at the very least, to have my unexposed film returned to me.

Curiously we find a new item in our car as a result of this crime. It's a black bowling ball zipped up in its own carrying case. This is beyond strange, but it might make sense from a criminal standpoint. Perhaps the thief hit another car earlier in the day and decided that, after looting our car, he didn't want the bowling ball after all. And so, in an act of untoward generosity, he left it with us. Unfortunately the damn thing is too small for my big hands and Deano doesn't want it either.

After a useless trip to the local police precinct, we're on the road out of Manhattan with a stiff wind to the backs of our heads and a bittersweet taste in our mouths. We stop in Center City Philadelphia, at the home of my aunt and uncle. My new plan is to stay here for a couple of days during which time I'll get the window fixed and install a new amplifier under my seat. Meanwhile, Deano catches a flight to Atlanta. The bill for the new glass will, once again, be sent to my father in Fort Lauderdale. Thankfully, this time the invoice is not followed by a round of psychiatric hospitalizations.

In November my Florida driver's license is set to expire, which means I have to get an Alabama license, since I'm now a state resident. I go to the license bureau in Opelika to fill out the required forms, and I see that there's a question on the application about having a history of mental illness. Not wanting to lie, I check the box marked YES.

This proves to be an error in judgment. The woman at the counter puts my application on hold, pending an interview by a sheriff. I drive away feeling defeated and demoralized with nothing to show for my efforts but an appointment for a police style mental status examination.

On the day of the appointment I do my best to make a good impression. I put on an ironed Oxford shirt and my finest pair of blue jeans—the ones without holes in the knees. A secretary points me to the sheriff's office, where I sit and wait a long time for him to show up. With nerves firing away, I look around the room at the plaques and the framed photos of cops posing in uniform. This is the land of the *good ole boy* network, meaning that anything I say must reflect well upon their ways. Flimsy thinking and liberal ideas won't cut it here. A deeply held respect for authority would serve me well. A Southern accent and references to Auburn Football and down home cooking might also help.

When the sheriff arrives, I feel more relaxed and ready to do the smooth talking. We shake hands. Then he asks a series of routine questions designed to determine whether my state of mind poses a hazard to the road. He lets me do most of the talking while he checks for flaws in my thinking. Above all else, I keep the ideas logically connected. When shifting from one thought to another, I make sure the segues are crystal clear. Logical reasoning is paramount. There can be no hint of loose association, not a speck of delusion, no morsel of paranoia, even though I'm paranoid of this cop revoking my driving privileges.

After about 30 minutes the sheriff acts like we're old friends. He signs the form allowing me to get my license, and he gives me a fraternal pat on the shoulder as we say our goodbyes. It's a small victory, yet the whole thing could have been avoided if only I'd checked the no box from the start.

Soon after the license ordeal I apply for a better paying job than the one I have with the entomology professor, which only pays minimum wage. I know a couple of students who work for the United Parcel Service where they make nine dollars an hour. They work about four hours a day before classes, loading and unloading delivery trucks. Except for the harsh pre-dawn starting time, I figure the job will be easy, especially with my experience at Van Arsdale's.

But I never make it past the application process. Just like the license bureau, UPS has this question about mental health history, and in my continued stupidity I answer the question honestly. I provide solid references and do all the things you're supposed to do for a job like that, but it's a wasted effort. A few weeks after filling out the forms, I call the office to check on my status only to hear a secretary tell me she has no such name on file. My guess is some UPS pencil pusher saw the box marked yes and tossed the application in the garbage. The message slowly sinks into my dense brain that honesty is not always the best policy.

So I continue to work at the professor's greenhouse, watering plants and picking cocoons for chicken-feed pay. To cut back on expenses, I eat the cheapest things I can find, like generic macaroni and cheese, canned tuna and—cheapest of all—ramen noodles for 12 cents a package.

Maybe it's good that I chose psychology as my future vocation. Surely the gatekeepers in this profession won't be so quick to condemn me for my past. The psychology professors here at Auburn show an open-minded view on most things. I tell one of them, Dr. Hess, about my earlier plight. When I finish the story, he looks proud of me and says my experiences could serve the field well. He knows the value of overcoming obstacles, and I judge his view as typical of the whole profession. I see psychology as an oasis, free from the harsh prejudices found in other areas of life. It makes sense that the admissions people at graduate programs would be equally open-minded.

As a senior with a high grade point average, glowing letters of recommendation, decent test scores and volunteer work at the crisis hotline, I figure my chances of getting into a doctoral program are pretty good. I've read the daunting statistics about how 90% of all applications are rejected, but this doesn't diminish my confidence. Just to be safe I fill out a couple of master's program applications in case all the doctoral programs reject me. Dr. Hess calls these "savior schools," but to me it would be a failure to take that route.

A key part of the doctoral application is the personal statement, which is an autobiographical essay ending with why you think you'd make a positive impact on the field of psychology. It's the only chance you get to be creative on the application and show how you stand apart from the pack. This is where I think I can shine. My riveting story of descent into madness, my struggle in the hospitals, my subsequent recovery, and my newfound sense of purpose is sure to be impressive. I write and rewrite the essay until I get it the way I like it. It recounts the crash, the struggle and the redemption, all in good balance. It ends on a triumphant note—three years without medication and no return to psychosis. With satisfaction I think my essay will give me an edge, and I'll be able to choose among the top programs.

But there's still a nagging sense of unease left from my experiences at the license bureau and UPS. It's something I don't yet understand, and it's the kind of lesson I have to get pounded in with a jackhammer before it sinks in. While I know it's good to stand apart from the pack, I don't realize yet that it's also a threat to stand too far from the pack. That's the role of the lone wolf, and such a creature isn't welcome in psychology or any other profession. The only way to be a lone wolf and still be accepted is to wear sheep's clothing. This I learn the hard way.

I apply to 10 doctoral programs, sending each the same personal statement with minor modifications, depending on how the question is framed. I wait with optimism once they're all sent out.

Soon the letters start arriving, each with the same formal tone. There's the concession of thanks, the *sorry to inform you...* and the *good luck in your future pursuits*. Not even a single interview is offered.

Thankfully there are the two master's programs I applied to, the savior schools, where a personal statement wasn't required and there were no boxes attached to questions about past mental health history. Both programs accept me, and one, Villanova University, offers a full tuition scholarship. With a mixture of frustration and relief, this is where I decide to go.

I have now learned a demoralizing lesson once and for all. If I ever fill out another form asking about psychiatric history,

I'll check the NO box. And next time around I'll write a different personal statement, watered down, with no mention of my psychotic past. It's like the lesson I learned after getting my ass kicked by DW in the sixth grade. *Hit him in the face! Deny your history!*

In the spring of '88 I graduate from Auburn with *cum laude* honors. I've gained a newfound confidence, ready to meet the challenges of Villanova. At the commencement ceremony in the packed Coliseum, I look up and see Phil and my family smiling and cheering from the bleachers. Their enthusiasm embarrasses me, but it's a good kind of embarrassment. The only disappointment of the day is my father. Just like my high school graduation, my dad doesn't make the trip. Some patterns are hard to break.

Graduation day is a joy with none of the reckless stupidity that characterized my exit from Cardinal Gibbons. And unlike my opinion of high school, I feel nothing but respect and gratitude for Auburn. This beautiful place has accommodated me through the best and the worst. There's magic happening here, and it's the kind of magic that can last a lifetime.

It's a curious phenomenon how a school can win over your heart so decisively. I don't think logic and reason can explain it. You could list hard facts about other schools having higher academic standards or prettier campuses, and it wouldn't have the slightest effect. It's an emotional thing really, and I'm under its spell. For me there will never be another Auburn.

29

M Y trip to Villanova in the summer of '88 is an eventful one. In Fort Lauderdale I rent a UHaul truck with an attached trailer for towing my car. After a little prodding, my 77-year-old grandmother agrees to accompany me on the long journey. Rhonda the cat, who's proven herself an excellent traveler, sits between my grandmother and me on the bench seat of the truck. Our plan is to drive back up to Auburn for the first leg of the trip. There we'll load up the furniture left in storage and add it to the stuff already onboard. From Auburn, it'll take another day and a half to get to Philadelphia's western suburbs. We're confident and ready for all possible hazards.

Yet the heat proves to be a hardship beyond what we expect. We're in the midst of one of the worst heat waves on record. To save money, I rented an old standard shift truck without air conditioning. The black vinyl seat is like a sweat-making factory, and there's no sense stopping to change clothes every hundred miles just to drench them too. A kind of heat induced misery settles upon all three of us.

Somewhere in Georgia, Rhonda starts panting with her tongue hanging out of her mouth. My grandmother strokes her forehead with ice cubes, and we keep the water bowl at Rhonda's chin. Instead of using the air vents for our minimal relief, we focus them on Rhonda, whose black fur must be cooking her insides. It's a painful thing to watch a cat suffer like this, but thankfully the water and the air vents help. I drive and curse the wicked heat, while my grandmother corrects my foul language and nurses Rhonda back to a state of vitality.

Relief for all comes when we reach a motel near the North Carolina border. The thick heat is still as oppressive as it's been all day, but the motel has air conditioning and an outdoor swimming pool.

Early next morning we prepare for the final leg of the trip. We eat breakfast at the motel's restaurant and pack our things in the truck. I put Rhonda in the truck cabin, then check the load in the cargo area. Everything looks fine. We're on schedule and ready to go. But then my grandmother asks where Rhonda is.

I check the cabin, which is where I thought I put her, but there's no sign of her. We double check to make sure, then we search all the places she might be. There's no sign of her anywhere.

Fear settles in as I run around the grounds of the motel, back into the motel room and any other place I can think of. We call out "Here Rhonda, Rhonda," and we make that lip-smacking sound to try and lure her back...but to no effect. I start feeling desperate, cursing the situation with foul language right in front of my grandmother. She tells me to stop the profanity and says I should re-check the truck cabin, which is where I swear I put her.

Lying on the floorboard of the truck, I reach my arm up into the guts of the dashboard, through a mess of wires and above the air ducts. Reaching farther still, I can feel a little clump of fur. "Holy shit" I say, and this time my grandmother doesn't scold me. With a little poking and pulling I get Rhonda to come down. When I see that she's okay, I give my grandmother a hug and apologize for the cussing. She forgives me, and in a few minutes we're back on the road contending with another day of heat.

Our destination is a Philadelphia suburb named King of Prussia, where I've secured a studio apartment. The only time I was there before was a confusing day during which my mother and I got lost trying to find the place. That was about a month ago. Now, with my young buck confidence on high, I figure I'll be able to find it with ease. I have the self-assurance that comes with driving a big truck cross-country, sitting up high, navigating with perfect accuracy. I have the necessary maps and an *X* on the desired location. No task is too big for me. At least that's my train of thought as we approach the exit ramp.

The Philadelphia suburbs have a way of dampening a person's navigational confidence. To speak of the tangled mess that constitutes this area is to do little justice to the true extent of it. You have to be in it to know the power of its misdirection. It happens as soon as you arrive. Exit the turnpike, pay your toll, and there before you is a confusing array of signs, merger lanes and nondescript buildings offering no directional clues. Here, every road curves and every community looks like the one before. Street names are duplicated with minor changes, like adding *Upper* or *Lower* to the name without any indication of what that means. Does upper mean direction, like north? Or maybe it means the road is on a hill? Or perhaps it leads to a community with the word Upper in it? To the uninitiated there's no telling.

We arrive late in the afternoon in heavy traffic with the skies an ominous gray. Negotiating lane changes is almost impossible with our slow moving truck and the car dragging behind. I'm supposed to turn right at Upper Gulph Road, but

I miss the turn and end up on a road I can't even find on the map. Undaunted, I make a couple of correction turns to get us back on track. This is my neighborhood now and I should know how to get around. Somehow, though, visualizing the way in my mind doesn't jibe with seeing it as it is. Soon it's clear that we're lost.

At an intersection I see a road with the name Gulph in it, so I think I should follow it. For that I need to make a U-turn. I pull into a hotel parking lot that looks like a good place to turn the truck. This turns out to be an act of poor planning. The parking lot is too narrow for a U-turn, but in my haste I try a three-point turn, which ends up being four or five points, each one making the situation more hopeless. Looking back, I see that the car, truck and trailer are an immovable, jackknifed mess, and we're blocking the way in and out of the parking lot.

Up to this point my grandmother has been the picture of stoicism, deferring to me and avoiding judgment. But now, stuck as we are like flies in a web, she speaks up. She tells me how we're not supposed to back up with the type of trailer we have. And as usual, she's right.

The most sensible strategy is to detach the car from the trailer and leave it here in the parking lot for later retrieval. So that's what I do. With a new sense of humility, I write down the name and location of the hotel in case I have a mild stroke between now and the time I come back for the car.

After re-examining the map, my grandmother and I are able to find the apartment complex without too much difficulty.

But now there's another problem. The property manager says my apartment isn't ready for occupancy yet, so I'll have to stay in a temporary apartment for the next two or three weeks. I'm not happy about this new twist, but what can I do? Then, as the property manager shows us my new short-term dwelling, the rain starts coming down hard. "Well, this is fucking great," I say in a soft voice, hoping my grandmother doesn't hear, but she does anyway. For now, she's given up correcting my language.

There's not much we can do at this point. With the heavy rain we can't unpack the truck. And though we're both hungry, neither of us wants to risk driving around in a loaded UHaul, looking for a restaurant and risking another episode of misdirection. The better option is for me to go back on foot to the hotel where I left my car.

I grab a chair off the truck for my grandmother and tell her I'll be back soon with the car. With map, keys and the hotel name stuffed in my pocket, I run off in a sprint, high-stepping through puddles.

Soon I realize that one of the problems with the suburbs is their lack of sidewalks, and the problem is compounded by rain. Running along the busy street, I get splashed repeatedly by passing cars. Since my grandmother isn't around, I can give full voice to the ugly language stored up inside me. Nothing is good. Everything sucks. I curse the rain and the drivers in their cozy, dry cars. I curse the street with its pothole puddles and no sidewalks. I curse the goddamn property manager and the goddamn fool who planned this vile suburban sprawl. I curse the mentality of the people who drive for miles and miles just to come here to goddamn King of Prussia, to shop at the fancy mall.

It's a tirade of cursing and dodging the splashing cars and puddles. After about a mile I'm drenched and worn out. With low expectations, I put my thumb out to hitch a ride. And, as I half expected, the cars zoom by, none of them stopping or even slowing down to consider a ride. There's a hardness in the way the drivers look when they pass. It's the same kind of hardness you see downtown when a pedestrian refuses to give a panhandler a quarter. There's no chance I'll be putting my wet ass in anyone's dry car today. I give up on the hitchhiking and walk on.

Maybe it's strange, but as I continue walking I give in to a new feeling of calm. The anger has wound itself down to nothing, and the entire day's crap dissipates into the unimportant. There's really nothing wrong at all. I'm safe. My grandmother and my cat are safe. Everything is fine, as it should be. It occurs to me that, except for the day in New York City when my car was burglarized, this was the angriest I've been since my incarceration in the hospital. And it didn't get the best of me. I can't help smiling at the thought of it.

In a couple of days my grandmother will be back in Florida, and I'll be starting a new life as a graduate student.

Prior to starting classes, I search for a part-time job to supplement my paltry income. I'll be getting a small stipend from the college as compensation for working six or seven hours a week on research projects. But the amount won't even be enough to pay my rent. I search the classified ads, looking for something where I can get paid while doing schoolwork.

My dad suggests working at a library, which is worth a shot, but then I see a listing for a night watchman at a retirement home, and it sounds like the job for me. The nurse who interviews me says the basic requirement is that I be a reliable "warm body," which means a living, breathing human being who's here when he's supposed to be. To this I say, "Yes, I can do the job."

The place is called Dunwoody Home, in Newtown Square, and I work the 11 P.M. to 7 A.M. shift where the obvious temptation is to sleep on the job. An empty bed on the first floor with crisp, white sheets calls my name. But if I go there, it's all over. They have this night watchman's clock with a keyhole in it to prove that I'm doing my job. Every hour I have to walk the length of the symmetrical building, from stairwell to stairwell, on both main floors and the basement.

The large colonial style structure was built in the early 20's, and the old keys hanging from chains along the walls are part of the original construction. There are 16 of them numbered throughout the facility, and my orders are to insert them into the night watchman's clock in proper sequence. Supposedly there's a ribbon of paper in there, which gets stamped with the time and date whenever I twist in a key. Looking through the keyhole, I can't tell whether the tape is actually in there—maybe it's only a ruse—but it's best to assume it's there anyway and that they actually check it regularly.

Other than twisting keys every hour, there's not much to do except for a few menial tasks to help the staff and residents get going in the morning. By far the most important of my duties is to make fresh coffee for the morning shift. If I forget to do this, I might as well haul my sorry ass out the building, never to return. To avoid such a scenario, I set my watch alarm for coffee making time and let no distractions interfere with this, the most sacred of obligations.

The psychology department at Villanova is housed in an old monastic style building, with laboratories, offices and small classrooms clustered in one wing of the U-shaped structure. Everything is packed into close quarters, which gives the place a sense of intimacy.

Classes here focus on the more scientific aspects of psychology, like statistics and experimental design, rather than on the art of conducting therapy or helping the downtrodden. If it came down to a battle between the art versus the science of psychology, science would win at Villanova, hands-down. It follows that the happiest students here are the ones who enjoy doing basic research, like my colleague Spencer who says his goal is to work with pigeons. When he shares this with me, I say something smart-ass like, "Hey, the skies the limit." It's hard for me to appreciate his passion for the bird, or for the bird's sensory-motor apparatus, or for its perceptual capabilities. It doesn't really interest me how long it takes a pigeon to learn how to peck at a lever to get food or avoid an electric shock. I don't see how this serves humanity or even the community of pigeons. At one point in 1984, I likened myself to a seagull, but I don't think Spencer would have anything positive to say about that, so I don't tell him.

The professor assigned as my mentor does basic research on a phenomenon known as the *Stroop Effect*. Here the participant is presented with several word lists he's supposed to read as fast as he can. The trick is that one of these lists has names of colors, such as *red* and *green* and *blue*, but the names are printed in opposing colors, like the word *red* printed in green ink. This creates mental interference, hampering the subject's reading speed compared to the other lists where there's no interference. That's the Stroop Effect, named after its creator, Dr. Stroop.

The first day or so that I learn about Stroop and his effect, I find it intriguing. And then, when I see it in action with myself and others, I think it's amusing, like a party trick. But the problem is that my professor—the guy I'm supposed to work with for the next two years—has a passion for the Stroop Effect bordering on obsession. He wants to know the cognitive mechanisms behind it, and he wants to set up experiments to help answer these riddles. As we talk, questions lead to more questions, such as whether males have more interference than females, or whether visually oriented people perform the task more slowly than those who are more sound oriented. Is it just a visual phenomenon? Or is it wrapped up in our cognitive expectations of how the world is supposed to work? And so on, ad nauseam.

As a good graduate student, I design an experiment to help tackle these questions, thus winning the favor of my professor. It's a study using students who are members of fraternities and sororities versus those who aren't. One list has words familiar to those in Greek organizations, such as *pledge*, *rush* and *haze*, which are printed in different colors. The students have to name the colors—not read the words—as fast as they can. I'm guessing that the Greeks will take longer because the words have a deeper connection for them, which will slow them down.

I'm proud of myself for coming up with such a neat little experiment, and my professor seems happy with his budding protégé. Maybe if we get positive results we can publish the study in a reputable journal with our names listed for posterity. Together, we'll transform the landscape of Stroop research for all time.

But it doesn't take long for me to get sick of the goddamn Stroop Effect, and I don't give a rat's ass about what's going on behind the cognitive curtain. As the days and weeks pass, it gets harder to go into the lab everyday and pretend I'm excited about something when I'm not. It's a good thing when I'm finished collecting data, and I no longer have to stopwatch spoiled undergraduates naming colors. Now it's a matter of plugging the data into a cumbersome statistical program.

A small measure of excitement returns when I send the data in for the final computations and await the results. But the feeling turns when everything comes up null—no effect, no journal article and no high praise from my professor. I go into his office full of gloom to give him the bad news.

Forever the scientist, his reaction is upbeat. He tells me that my little study can be part of a set of experiments designed to more thoroughly uncover what's going on with the Stroop Effect. He starts up another conversation about the mediators behind the phenomenon and how my results could give us a clue as to what's really happening. I say nothing, but inside I can feel the life force fading away.

Returning to my apartment after the day's failure, I hit the play button on my phone machine. There's a message from Rhonda's veterinarian, stating that my cat died today in surgery. She was scratched a few weeks ago by another cat, which led to an infection that never healed. Now she's dead, and I have to pay for the failed surgery and the burial fee. I sit on the floor of my lonely apartment filled with tears and anger. The feelings stay with me throughout the evening and through the night shift at the retirement home.

I find out from my mother that Dunwoody Home is the same place where my great-grandfather spent the final years of his life. He was a German-born musician who played percussion for the Philadelphia Orchestra before going a little senile in the early 1960's, thus warranting his final place of residence. My mother said he died at the age of 90, about two weeks after I was born. With a little investigation, I figure out which room was his.

My great-grandfather's old room is at the north end of the hall on the second floor. It's now the place where an unkempt crazy man named Fred lives. He usually stays up well into the wee hours, drinking coffee, pacing the halls and, when the mood strikes, yelling out a stream of violent babble. One night I knock on Fred's door, and when he answers I tell him that my great-grandfather used to live in this very place. I expect Fred to be flattered by the connection. But instead he looks at me with a serious face and says, "Your soul is blacker than black!"

It's a tough thing to hear, especially coming from Fred, who I've grown to like. I want to know what he means and whether there's any logic in how he came up with his assertion. But I'm paralyzed by the words themselves. I think of when I used to say such things in the hospital and how I still think there was a grain of truth in most of it. Backing away from his room, I consider the alleged blackness of my soul. To shake off the feeling, I pace the halls of Dunwoody, just as I did at Fort Lauderdale Hospital.

The next morning, once the staff arrives, I tell the head nurse what happened with Fred. She says he's a chronic schizophrenic who's been in and out of several hospitals and he's been taking Prolixin for decades. She says he's been a lot worse than he was last night, and I should just get used to it.

The ordeal with Fred makes me think about my own predicament and how I could've ended up like him. A wave of sadness comes over as I drive home in the morning rush hour. The sadness is for me and also for Fred.

A couple of nights later, I go back to his room to give it another try. This time he's altogether different, and he invites me in, remembering why I came to his room in the first place. He says I should come in and see what he's done to my great-grandfather's old room.

I'm shocked at the change and happy to have the old Fred back. My soul doesn't feel quite so black tonight.

While in his room, I try to imagine my great-grandfather speaking in nonsensical German about his glory days in the orchestra. It gives me a hollow feeling, and I don't stay there very long. Fred has these pin-ups of sexy women on his walls, which take me out of the moment. It's difficult to conjure up the spirit of your great-grandfather when there are naked women posing at you.

The closest I come to rejuvenating his spirit is through my vigorous walks up and down the long halls with my Walkman, blasting Sinead O'Connor. I make like I'm playing the drums while the song *Jerusalem* bangs away in my head. Despite the late hour, I feel as alive as I've ever been. Maybe this is the way the old man felt when he walked these same halls.

The saddest night at Dunwoody Home is Christmas Eve, 1988. As the new guy on the job, I get stuck working the holiday instead of spending it down in Fort Lauderdale with my family. My mother sent me a huge brown box with a bunch of wrapped gifts inside from her and my sisters. I brought it with me tonight. At around midnight, after the first round with the night watchman's clock, I sit at the front desk and call home.

Soon it's a three-way conversation with my mother and Julia on the other end. I've got the phone clamped between my ear and shoulder while I'm tearing open the boxes and saying complimentary things about the new gifts.

"I wish you could be here," says Julia in a weepy voice.

I feel the sadness of it welling up, and I try to say the same thing back. Only I can't get the words out without crying a little bit. Then Julia cries, and then my mother cries, and now it's a big crying jag of a Christmas. Next year, I promise I'll be home for the holiday.

30

I T's the start of my second year at Villanova, and there's a new crop of graduate students here getting acclimated to their new environment. I like to hear them talk enthusiastically about psychology and their hopes of making an impact on the world. They'll find out soon enough that their dream of helping the mentally ill won't be addressed here, at least not during their first year. But I don't want to say anything cynical just yet.

One of these new students named Beth has captured my attention above all others. She's beautiful in all the ways a woman could be, at least physically so. I try to look at her without staring because the temptation to stare is ever-present. I feel like a salivating pervert whenever I'm near her.

Despite the fact that my brain is lost in sexual fantasy, my goal is to appear intelligent when I'm around Beth, like a wise elder student. But God, what a sexy thing she is! She looks like Paula Abdul, only a bit taller, and she carries herself like an erotic dancer. She can dance for me anytime, day or night.

As it turns out, Beth has been eyeing me too, which is

something I find out through my friend Rob at a bar. We've been drinking for hours with a bunch of other students, and as the alcohol consumption increases so does the truth telling. I don't catch what Beth says, but Rob, with his greater clarity of mind, does. He tells me about it when we're alone in the bathroom. "Man, that Beth chick has the hots for you!" he says.

I can't imagine sweeter words.

As the party breaks up, I offer to give Beth a ride home. She accepts and smiles with a wink. When we arrive at her building, she invites me up for a tour of her apartment. Then at the threshold of her door, she yawns and goes to lie down on her couch, making room for me. Not requiring a written invitation, I snuggle into the couch alongside her, and I work up the nerve to kiss her. With the TV turned to an old Barbara Streisand movie, Beth drifts into sleep. I get up to leave, and she awakens, promising she'll be more lively the next time we get together.

One thing about dating Beth that I hadn't fully anticipated is the effect she has of draining my already miniscule bank account. It's not her fault really. It's just that she's beautiful and extravagant, and she likes extravagant things. I'm too weak to resist her charms, which becomes an expensive flaw for a struggling graduate student. My credit card only makes the situation worse. Every time we go out, I charge it on the card with no idea of when I'll be able to pay it off. I think it's worth it because she's so beautiful and because she likes me.

Near the end of the fall semester, I'm thinking seriously about dropping out of Villanova. As much as I would like to have my master's diploma in hand, I realize it isn't necessary for getting into a doctoral program. If I stay, I'll have to work extra hard on my thesis, and I haven't even selected a topic yet. Most students don't finish their theses in the two years anyway, and these are people who actually like what they're doing. With my motivation at an all-time low, there's no way I'll finish in time. And the longer I stay the deeper I get into debt.

The best way out, as far as I can see, is to get a full-time job with decent pay. I'll quit Villanova and the Dunwoody Home as soon as I find a replacement job, and I'll work regular hours like a regular guy. That'll be a blessed change from the night shift and my screwed up sleep cycle. Plus, with a steady job I can live it up a little without getting swallowed by debt. Dollar signs are prancing in my brain.

I want a job in the mental health field where I can work with patients and find out what it's like to be on the other side. It's been four and a half years since my imprisonment at Fort Lauderdale Hospital, but the place still has a grip on me. It feels as though they took something away from me, and I want it back. What they took, I'm not exactly sure, but hopefully I can find out by working in a similar place. I'm excited and scared at the same time.

There's a job opening for a psychiatric aide at a private hospital. It bears the impressive name Northwestern Institute, located in Fort Washington, which is about a 20 minute commute through a chunk of the suburban maze. After a short interview and a background check, I'm offered the job.

My title is an ambiguous thing, even to the staff of the hospital. I don't know whether to refer to myself as an attendant, an aide, a psychiatric technician or an orderly. I've been hired along with five other people, and together we go through a weeklong training process. We learn the rules and the logistics of the building, crisis intervention and communication skills with the patients. We do role-playing exercises to test our new-found skills, and we all feel confident and ready to tackle the job when the training is over. It occurs to me that there isn't a single thing I learned at Villanova that would be of use here. This is the clinical realm, and it's a galaxy apart from the realm of basic research. If I mention Stroop, they'd look at me like I'm from a different planet.

Throughout my training and the first few weeks on the job, I feel like a fraud. For one thing, I told the kindly woman who hired me that I consider this a permanent arrangement. For another, my now standard lie of omission was to tell her nothing about my history of being a patient in a place like this. Of course, if I had told her the truth I never would have landed this job.

After a few weeks I figure the staff is no worse off for their ignorance of these facts, and I doubt the patients would care either way. Sometimes lying to get ahead in life is the way it has to be. Being here day after day, collecting a regular paycheck is proof that the lying paid off.

Most days I work the evening shift from 3 to 11 P.M., but occasionally we're short-staffed, so I'm forced to work a double shift whether I like it or not. It's good for the wallet, with time-and-a-half pay, but I pay for it with exhaustion the next day.

The job primarily involves sitting and watching patients and writing notes in their charts about whether they're behaving appropriately or not. Some days I sit in on group therapy, and other days I help run volleyball games in the gym.

There's an art therapy group where patients are making ceramic sculptures, and I have to sit in and keep watch on some of the more difficult cases. I have to be on the lookout for an *escalation of inappropriate behavior*, perhaps culminating in the use of clay as weaponry. Things could get ugly.

While on watch, I also get to make my own piece of sculpture. I make a bowl with decorative etchings all around and a happy face in the inside center for comic effect. At first I don't care much for it, just going through the motions. But soon I become transfixed by the project and how it's progressing. When the group is over I want to stay and finish my bowl, but I can't because I have to escort patients back to the unit and make sure they don't run off or kill themselves.

In the evening I sneak back to the art therapy room to retrieve my bowl. While on break at the nurse's station, I sit and work on it again, adding a ribbon of clay around the lip. When it's dry, I paint it with an assortment of colors, mostly greens and blues. Then it's sent to the kiln with a batch of other stuff made by patients.

A week or so later my bowl comes back, and I'm proud of it—my first bowl. To me, it's the best bowl in all of Northwestern Institute. Like a kid at show-and-tell, I let others hold it and tell them I'm giving it to my girlfriend Beth. Of course they say she'll like it very much.

When I present it to Beth, she says, "Hey it's really cute." Then she puts the bowl on her bookshelf, where she'll use it to store bobby pins.

From her bed I look across the room at the once proud bowl, and I'm hurt by the apparent neglect. I imagine eating a hearty helping of beef stew out of it. That would do it justice, honoring the effort that went into it. But a gift is a gift, and in this case it's a dust trap. Next bowl I'm keeping for myself.

There are times on the job when I have to play a part in restraining unruly patients, and it's a strange feeling being on the other side like this. No matter how bad they get with their screaming fits, name calling and attempts to knock me out, I don't feel angry in the slightest. Other things piss me off for sure. If a driver on the highway cuts me off, I'm the first to extend my middle finger in a tirade of cussing. Here in the hospital, though, it's a sad thing to restrain patients against their will. It's sadder still when the nurse comes in with the goddamn syringe and plunges some poor soul into helplessness and sleep. The anger I have is reserved for the system—for the shrink who wrote the prescription and for the nurse who's only following orders. Then again, I'm also following orders. I keep watch over the ordeal and say nothing. Like the patient, I have to hold back my true feelings.

Inside I'm filled with a mixture of reactions, and I wonder if there isn't a better way. Just like me in '84, these patients don't know what they're in for once they get here. Maybe they think this is a place where they can rest and take a much needed break from the stress of life. Ideally, this could be a place where they're allowed to go crazy, to let it out, to scream in a sound-proof chamber for a while. They could knock around dummies in a rubber room, all with the guidance of a supportive staff. That would be a godsend to some of these people.

But the reality is that these patients are caught in a web of social control and chemical manipulation. Like all psychiatric wards, this is a place where the combined forces of medical psychiatry, the pharmaceutical industry, insurance companies and state government all work in collusion to force patients into obedience. Failure to comply is addressed through the use of restraints, both chemical and physical. Once these are exhausted, court orders can then be employed. As a result, these patients learn to hide their demons, as I did—forcing them underground where they grow into a darker and more sinister force. This leads to the application of more drugs and longer stays in the hospital. It's no wonder that many of them become crippled for life. Worse yet is the fact that few people seem to care. The shrinks, the nurses, the support staff and the administration all play these mindless roles without considering alternatives. And the patients' families don't know enough to demand some form of change.

A few months into my employment, I get the unusual assignment of working on the all-female unit for personality disorders, including the controversial diagnosis of multiple personality disorder. It's a strange scene watching a woman shift from one personality—for example, a defiant boy—to something totally different. The change looks real enough to me, and it makes sense when one of the nurses tries to explain it. She says these are intelligent and creative women who formed these personalities to insulate themselves from the torment of being molested years ago. She goes on to say that everyone has a signature way of dealing with traumatic stress, and this is their signature. Only now they're stuck in the past, and they're stuck with a twisted way of dealing with everyday life. To fix the problem is like trying to reconstruct Humpty Dumpty.

The majority of the other women on the unit have the vague sounding diagnosis of borderline personality disorder, which is supposed to mean that they're on the border between neurotic and psychotic with components of each. These patients show such a messy array of symptoms that I'm left exasperated when I try to help them. One moment they're sweet to me, saying provocative and pleasant things. Then the next moment I'm the ally of Satan himself.

A key reason why many of these women landed themselves here is because they mutilated themselves, usually by burning or cutting their skin with a knife. They say they do it not so much out of self-hatred or to kill themselves, but because they like the release that the pain itself gives them. As I hear this, I'm also thinking that they must like the attention they get from it. I mean, how do you ignore someone sitting there putting out cigarettes on her forearm?

A good number of the women on the unit are obese, and some talk about the origins of their weight problem. Several say that the added girth is to cover the pain of their existence. Most of them wear bulky sweaters, even when it's hot out, so that no one can see their shape and fantasize about them sexually. They associate sex with pain and rage, so it's better to hide under their bulk.

But then there are others who dress like whores on the

prowl. One such woman propositions me, and when she doesn't like what I say back to her, she lets loose with a firestorm of rage. I swear to the nurse that I didn't do anything. The nurse's response is, "You're a man. That's enough." Worse yet, I'm the only man on the unit, so I take the heat for all men.

To me the whole thing is a confusing, toxic mess, and I don't want to stay the whole eight hour shift. I sit slouched in a corner with my clipboard and my raw nerves, hoping no one notices me. I wonder if I did something to piss off the scheduling supervisor who assigned me to work here in this unit of the hospital for three consecutive days. My plan is to do nothing but sit and try to avoid setting someone off.

As I consider the burden of being here, I also remember something that happened to me when I was five years old. It's a dark memory, no doubt triggered by my current circumstances, and it comes back to my brain like it was yesterday.

It happened when we lived in Pompano Beach, before my parents split up. Two friends and I were exploring a construction site where they were building a house in one of the few remaining open lots. It was exciting to see the cement trucks drive up and pour out the slab. Then other trucks came to deliver mounds of cinder blocks and bags of cement mix stacked on pallets. After the workers went home for the day, we played around in the dirt and found sticks to use as swords.

One afternoon a girl named Paula caught us running around the site with our sticks. She came over and told us we aren't allowed to be here. She warned us about trespassing on private property and, because she was older and bigger than we were, she could force us to leave.

My friends and I lacked the will to put up a fight, so we started for the street. But then we saw Paula climbing up to the top of a stack of cement bags. When she got to the top, she stood there proud, like she was the queen of Egypt or something. She started taunting us, saying how she was so much stronger and smarter and faster. It went on for some time, and we yelled back at her, but our words sounded feeble next to hers. When she grew tired of the taunting, she signaled me out of the group and dared me to climb up and join her.

Ashamed of being outdone by Paula, I hoped that by climbing up I could re-establish some pride. So I wedged my fingers and sneakers into the cracks between the cement bags and slowly made my way up. As I did this, she renewed her taunting, this time telling my friends how weak and how slow I was and how I'd never make it to the top.

Eventually, though, I made it all the way up. I smiled at my buddies from on high. It was a brief moment of glory. As soon as I turned my back to Paula, she kicked me hard in the butt, letting out a grunt as I went belly-flop style onto the ground. The impact knocked the wind out of me, and the pain was severe. Blood dribbled from my forehead onto the gravel. I cried as hard as a boy of five cries, which made Paula laugh and call me a crybaby. She sang, "Crybaby, crybaby, you're just a crybaby."

I yelled back with a thin voice, while my friends picked me up and carried me down the street to my house.

My mother was frantic when she saw her bloody mess of a son. She lifted me onto the kitchen counter, set my head in the sink and pointed the faucet over my forehead. She flushed out the dirt with water and checked my body for other scrapes. She focused on the spot just above my right eye. That's where the stitches would go. My mother said I was lucky not to have damaged the eye. But lucky wasn't how I felt. While driving to the hospital, she said, "That Paula girl is sick in the head," which didn't mean much to my five-year-old brain.

I wanted to get back at Paula and plotted all sorts of ways to do it. But I knew I could never go through with the plans. Paula was stronger, smarter and more sadistic. And, unlike me, she had the stomach to carry out whatever she wanted to do. If

I took action, she'd match it and then add on another retaliatory step with pleasure. I would be no contest for the likes of her. The best thing was to avoid her.

Thus, instead of a crybaby, I became a "scaredy-cat" whenever Paula was around. Soon thereafter, we moved to our new house in Fort Lauderdale, and I never saw her again.

In light of my experience with Paula, I can understand why the taunting of these women on the unit unnerves me as much at it does. I also understand a little better why I obeyed Danny's idiotic directive back on the last day of high school. The sensible thing would have been to say, "No Danny, that's ridiculous," and drive on. But maybe part of my obedience was pent-up Paula rage surfacing out of a drunken stupor. And maybe that's why now, with these disturbed women jerking me back and forth, it feels like Paula revisited, like I'm five and helpless again. The thought of it gives me a chill.

With these thoughts playing in my mind, the charge nurse comes over to tell me that I have to sit in on a music therapy session. The group will include the eight women from the unit considered to be the most stable. They're allowed off the floor for group activity, but they still need supervision. Leading the group will be a gay male therapist.

We gather in a small room with the chairs set up in a circle. The room is too small for me to play the invisible man. I have to sit in the circle and act calm, like I can handle any crisis they throw at me. The therapist starts with group discussion, asking the women about what's holding them back from recovery.

First there's a strained silence, but then one of the more vocal patients jumps in with a speech about how she was raped by her stepfather. It's an angry and dramatic story and, by the end of it, the energy of the room has shifted. Her story is followed by a series of similar accounts of victimization, each telling of abuse by bad men. These are war stories, and it's the same oppressor every time—the bad straight male.

The gay therapist is immune from evil glances, but I'm not so lucky, and I feel like a creep even though I didn't do anything. If I tell them about Paula, I might get some sympathy. But if I talk about Lois and her bicycle, I'll be the target of fresh rage. It's best to shut up and look sincere.

After the tragic stories are dredged up, the therapist changes focus. He asks us to close our eyes and relax, telling us to concentrate on our breathing. We do as instructed, and the room is quiet for a moment. Then there's the sound of the therapist fumbling with a tape deck. He gets it cued up, and we can hear soft music. Right away, I can tell it's the song *Wind beneath My Wings*, by Bette Midler. At first I don't know why he's playing this song—I'm looking for a logical segue—but soon I can see the genius of it. Automatic catharsis is his aim, and it works like a switch.

As Bette sings, "Did you ever know that you're my hero…?" one of the first women to tell her story breaks into a sob. Then a couple of others follow with a bigger outpouring of tears. Soon the whole group turns into a wet mess, and this genius of a therapist has a fresh box of Kleenex to pass around.

I feel guilty as I pass the box without taking a tissue because I haven't been crying. It's no fault of Bette Midler's. It's just that I'm not in the mood. If I cried about anything, I think I'd cry about the five-year-old boy I once was—the dumb kid who had no idea what he was in for. God bless him.

After my shift is over at eleven o'clock, I drive over to Beth's apartment to decompress. I don't say much about the day. Instead, we sit on the floor by the foot of her bed. She seems to know that I only want to sit here and hold her, and let her hold me.

31

EARLY in the spring of 1990 I'm preparing myself to interview for doctoral programs in clinical psychology. As I look over a slew of brochures, one place stands out as my favorite. It's the one at Indiana State University, and it sounds great on paper. Their training emphasis is on therapy and patient intervention over research, and I figure the cost of living in Terre Haute, Indiana, is probably a lot less than I pay here. I've heard horror stories about graduate students going deep into debt—mortgage size debt—to pay for their years in school. Once they finish, they're stuck with an obnoxious monthly payment for a good chunk of their careers. It gets to the point where they resent ever having gone to graduate school in the first place. I don't want to go down that road, so I look for places that won't pauperize me.

As I sit through the idle hours at work, guarding a sedated patient, I read the ISU program brochure and study the map of Terre Haute sent over by the Chamber of Commerce. I examine the orderly grid of streets on the map, the shaded box downtown representing the college, the wavy blue line representing the Wabash River, and I imagine how it might look in reality. My mind buzzes with clean, colorful images of Terre Haute—centerpiece of America's heartland—and I'm in the scene of my imagination, walking from my downtown apartment to class, then to an urban café where I have lively discussions about life and psychology with my new colleagues.

With almost zero knowledge of the Midwest, I pull from a few familiar sources to create the scenes in my brain. The result is a hodgepodge of Auburn, Philadelphia and the movie *Field of Dreams* with endless tracts of corn and noble men. The only true thing I know about Indiana State is that Larry Bird went there, and he put the place on the map of college basketball glory for a fleeting moment.

In addition to the map and brochure, I also have a letter from the ISU psychology department offering me an interview. Going there in person is the wise thing to do, I know, but that would be expensive, and I don't have enough vacation or sick time accrued at work. I decide to take a telephone interview instead.

My interview is scheduled for nine o'clock tomorrow morning with a Dr. Krugman. With 12 hours to go before the phone call, I'm confident I'll be ready to make a good impression.

But Northwestern Institute won't make it easy for me. The hefty nursing supervisor tracks me down to tell me I have to work a double shift because one of the regular night staff workers called in sick. At first I say, "No I can't do it," going on about an important meeting I have. Of course, I can't say what that meeting is.

But it doesn't matter. The portly nurse says, "If you don't do the double shift, you'll be fired, simple as that."

I want to tell her she can take my fucking timecard and shove it up her fat ass, but I need the money too much. It's a shame I never get to say anything like that.

So I do the double shift, and by 7 A.M. I'm a bleary-eyed, sluggish mess. As quickly as possible, I race back to King of Prussia in a sea of well-rested commuters on their way to work. Once home, I doze off for about an hour. The alarm clock is set for 8:30, and when it goes off I think it's the most obnoxious sounding thing ever created. It's not a thought I dwell on. I have exactly 30 minutes to rouse myself from irritable stupor into prime candidate material.

I become a storm of activity—making strong coffee, splashing cold water on my face, testing out my vocal chords with loud expletives while pacing back and forth in the small apartment between sips of coffee.

At nine o'clock the phone rings, and it's Dr. Krugman. He tells me a few basic things about the program, and I let him know how interested I am. Then he presses onward with the interview questions.

Somewhere in the midst of my delirium, I explain about the double shift and my struggle not to slur my words, and Dr. Krugman laughs a little. That's a good sign. He becomes friendlier, and he tells me that he knows people in Philadelphia, which is a very good sign. Geographic bonus points—a big plus! The rest of the interview is lost to the recesses of my sleep deprived memory.

About a month later, I'm accepted into the program. "Jesus, that was easy," I say to myself. What's the catch?

The catch, if you can call it that, is really two things: Terre Haute, Indiana, and the college itself. Sight unseen, they both look great, especially with the favorable workings of imagination. I find out otherwise when Beth and I take a road trip there to search for an apartment.

We pick what must be the hottest four day stretch of the summer. It's the kind of weather where you sweat in the brief moment of walking from air-conditioned car to air-conditioned building. To get an apartment without A/C would be a case of true masochism. A couple of townspeople tell us the real meaning of Terre Haute is *Terrible Hot*, and they laugh at their own wit. I can tell they've probably laughed at this piece of nonsense a hundred times before.

Apartment hunting is a chore. There's nothing decent downtown—just shabby old houses subdivided into shabby little apartments. We comb the paper and make phone calls, looking at one shit-hole of an apartment after another. Finally, I end up with a place on the northern periphery of town where my backyard adjoins a large soybean field.

With the remaining balance of time, Beth and I ride around looking for the good qualities of the town and college. On days like this, with the paper factory operating at full velocity, the smell is an overpowering sensory assault. The only good thing I can say about this is that you could fart and no one would notice the difference.

Driving along the main north-south route, you can't help but notice the motel bearing the name and face of Larry Bird. Once inside, you find the image of Bird's face on almost everything, including the shower curtains. If there's such a thing as a patron saint of Terre Haute, Bird is it. If I had a vote on the matter, my choice would be Theodore Dreiser, author of *Sister Carrie* and *American Tragedy*, but no one here seems to know about old Dreiser.

Terre Haute doesn't exactly stand for high culture, or *haute couture*, as Beth says. I don't really care about its lack of fine restaurants, museums or specialty shops. But the vacant stores, the ugliness of the campus and the flatness of the region do bother me. It seems easy, almost automatic, to develop a hatred for Terre Haute and the surrounding community. It's not so easy learning to like it. That would take time and a willing spirit.

❀

By summer's end, things aren't going so well between Beth and me. It starts and ends with the fact that she cheated on me, and there's no easy fix for that. I know she doesn't want to live in Terre Haute either, and who could blame her? I think she'd resent me for dragging her out there, and maybe she resents me now for the prospect of it. I wonder if that's why she cheated.

It's pointless to mull it over, and in a way it's a blessing. I can start my new life without the strain of a long-distance relationship. It's exciting to move forward and advance my goals without any attachments, free to move on to new and inspiring possibilities.

Still, I know I'll miss Beth.

32

I N Terre Haute, I fill the void of losing Beth by spending time with the other graduate students, especially my assigned *buddy*, Annette. She's a year ahead of me in the program, and she drew my name from among the batch of incoming students to help me get acclimated. Annette is a large, noble looking black woman from the University of Maryland. I'm not physically attracted to her, so there's nothing sexual between us. I don't know how the other assigned buddies act, but Annette seems to take her role seriously. She calls at least two or three times during the week before classes start, and she continues to call and visit after we're well into the semester. Maybe she wants to make sure I'm psychologically ready for the rigors of ISU. Or maybe she's just lonely, which is okay because I'm lonely too.

Eventually Annette and I develop a strong friendship, even after her buddy commitment expires. It's the first time I have a female friend, who's a real friend, without sex getting in the way. The best times Annette and I have together are our walks around Collette Park. We pace the interior road, circling round and round, talking nonstop into the late night hours. It's an energizing thing, as if everything we say means something. We cover all topics, except for superficial chitchat about the weather and such. Football is another subject Annette wants nothing to do with. She doesn't care about how the Auburn Tigers played in today's game. If the team loses, I can't help but vent my anger. Annette gives me a funny look and says, "Let it go."

Instead of football, we talk about life and how we think the world should change. We plunge into the topics of literature, politics, spirituality and even psychology. Sometimes we confront each other about the so-called psychological baggage we each carry around with us, and sometimes the confrontations get heated. For a time, Annette is the only person in the State of Indiana who knows about my life in the wacko wards of 1984. Like others before her, she says it could become a valuable asset someday.

"I don't know," I say and let the subject pass.

Part of my responsibility at ISU, as it was at Villanova, is to work with an assigned professor. Mine is Dr. Cerny, whose research consists of studying the human male sexual response. It's an area that might be of interest to me, since I am male and I have a sexual response. It must be more interesting than the Stroop Effect.

A colleague, Todd, is also part of the research team. Together, we're supposed to get willing participants, in the form of male undergraduates, to sit naked from the waist down and watch porno films. Attached to their penises is a vibrating device called a plethysmograph, which we refer to as the *peter meter*. The participants have control over the frequency of vibrations during the film, and they're able to rate how much they like or dislike the film. Data showing vibration frequency and penile blood flow are sent to a computer for later analysis. The printer pumps out a stream of coordinates showing a steady ascent in all physiological measures until *blast off*—ejaculation—followed by a precipitous drop in arousal.

Dr. Cerny's lab is in the basement of Root Hall, below the psychology department and away from potential voyeurs. I certainly don't want to watch the penises going up and down, and I don't think Todd does either, but I'm not so sure about the professor. After getting coached on the procedure, I want to know why we're doing this. My training at Villanova taught me to ask: what research hypotheses are we investigating? I want a coherent answer, and when I don't get one, my distrust of authority is activated. I wonder whether we're dealing with a sick pervert.

First opportunity available, I switch to a different professor. Now I work with Dr. Nelson, who teaches classes on personality theory. My job is to substitute teach and grade papers. I've traded in the peter meter for a red pen, and I'm happy about the change.

The program at ISU strongly emphasizes psychological testing, and it provides excellent training if that's where your interests lie. In the first year of the program, we learn about the different types of IQ tests, achievement tests and personality tests. We learn the meaning of the test scores and how the tests were originally constructed. Then we go out and use our skills on human subjects, and we test, and we test again. We compute the numerical scores under the pretext that they give us the story of the test taker.

With data in hand, we type up a carefully worded report with several different sections, the most important of which is called TEST RESULTS AND INTERPRETATION. Here's where the skill of the psychologist really comes into play. Armed with these data, we size up the person while trying not to give too much weight to our own personal biases.

Distilling the structure of personality and intelligence through test data and the clinical interview is the central magic of being a clinical psychologist. This is what separates us from psychiatrists (who medicate) and social workers (who counsel and organize services). But what are we supposed to do once our report is complete and we've finished our analysis of the patient?

This is where things get murky. Some recommend using psychotherapy alone to treat problems. Some advise medication. Most promote a combination of therapy and drugs. We leave it to the psychiatrists to choose the type of drug, although this is beginning to change as psychologists lobby for prescription authority. When it comes to selecting a certain type of therapy, we do have our biases, which often means choosing the style of therapy that we're most comfortable with, as long as it's covered by the patient's health insurance. Examples may include cognitive-behavioral, psychodynamic, humanistic or primal screaming in the woods. A new type of therapy seems to crop up every year or so. Science lags behind.

At times I wonder whether I really want to be a psychologist. Most people in the department seem so stiff and phony all the time, and I hate dressing up with a tie when I see patients in the clinic. The name of the game here is *impression management*. Keep them thinking that you're doing great, humming along, learning important things and always making meaningful progress. It's the look of calm, self-composed confidence. I know the look from my days in the hospital, and I know how to play this game. But I wonder if it's worth it.

Away from the psychology department, I need to find some balance, some counter-opposing force to inoculate me from the four year head trip and the fifth year internship. I can tell the program is already taking its toll because I'm not sleeping some nights, and my lower back feels like a severed nerve.

My dad is a good one to call at times like this. He's been through medical school and knows about the sucking up required to get through. I tell him I'm thinking of buying a motorcycle for touring around the area, and I wonder aloud about how much it might cost. Before the week is out, there's a check in the mailbox for a thousand dollars. And I haven't even picked out a bike yet.

I find what seems like the perfect motorcycle. It starts with me telling a colleague, Marlene, about my wish to find one. She tells her husband on the phone about it, and the secretary at his office overhears the conversation. The secretary's husband owns an old motorcycle, which he hasn't ridden in over four years, and she wants him to get rid of it. To her it's just wasting space in their garage.

A day later, I'm on the phone with the secretary talking about the bike and her husband. She tells me he's a retired coal-miner afflicted with a bad case of black lung. The motorcycle is a black 1977 Honda 750 with a fiberglass fairing and a luggage rack on the back. It has just over 4,000 miles on it, and the price is $750—one dollar per cubic centimeter of displacement. Without even looking the thing over, I tell her I want it.

The next day I pay a visit to Mr. John Doyle, owner of the motorcycle. His wife answers the door and takes me to her husband's bedroom where there's an assortment of inhalers and medicine bottles lined up next to a Lay-Z-Boy chair. The man sits in the recliner with a clear tube draped across his face, which is attached to a loud machine pumping out oxygen. In his hand is the remote control for the TV. He's watching a program about birds or hunting with the volume turned way up.

Mr. Doyle is a short heavy-set man with a white T-shirt snug against his beer belly. His voice is raspy and thick with mucous. His wife says he's having a bad day today, but he insists otherwise. He speaks in short segments, like an old en-

gine gasping on fumes. He gets frustrated with himself, cursing up and down, then he says to me, "Christ Almighty, don't
smoke and don't work in a goddamn coal mine."

I tell him I don't smoke, and I say that I'm a graduate student, but I don't tell him I'm studying psychology because
I'm afraid he'll think I'm one of those soft liberals. I can tell
Mr. Doyle doesn't want any soft liberals riding around on his
motorcycle.

It's an ordeal for him to get up out of his chair and even
harder for him to walk out to the garage with his oxygen can-
ister rolling behind. But we make it, and my heart starts racing
when I first see the bike. It's covered in dust, and the tires are
nearly flat. Cobwebs span the spokes, and there are larger spi-
der webs draped throughout the frame, engine and tailpipes.

"She's a little dirty, but once you get her going, she'll run
like a top," Mr. Doyle explains. "This here's a real motorcycle—not like one of them damn crotch rockets."

With every word I'm afraid his lungs might collapse, so
I try to keep him from long-winded conversation. He's not
much of a talker anyway, but he's proud of his bike. He says he
keeps thinking he'll be able to ride it again. I think snowballs
in hell are more likely.

Over the span of a week's worth of afternoons, Mr. Doyle
and I work on the bike until she's ready to ride. We put the
battery on a trickle charger, and I try to inflate the tires with
a feeble hand pump. The throttle won't turn because the bar
connecting the four carburetors is seized up with gunk. I have
to take the gas tank off and manually turn the throttle bar with
a vise grip to get it loose.

Another problem is the old gas in the carburetors, which I
guess has been sitting there for four years or more. I drain the
tank and spray the carburetors with cleaner, but it doesn't do
much good. I'll have to take them apart and clean each manually. It's a chore, but it's a good way to get familiar with the

bike.

By the end of it, John Doyle and I are like old friends. He gives me some extra things he'll never use again, like an old helmet, a shop manual, waxes, extra light bulbs and straps for holding down luggage. I pay him the $750 and thank him for the extra stuff. Without a trace of sentimentality, Mr. Doyle says, "Drive safe, and come back and visit." I beep the horn as I head out the back alley.

Once on the road, I realize this bike isn't safe to drive. For one thing, the old tires are badly under-inflated and the sidewalls cracked. I pull over at a gas station to inflate the tires, hoping the old things don't burst.

It occurs to me that something doesn't sound right. Soon I realize that the number three cylinder isn't firing. I can tell by spitting on the exhaust pipes and seeing that my spit doesn't melt away on the third pipe.

Hobbling to my house on Maple Avenue, I also realize that the seat is a torture chamber. Since Mr. Doyle is short, he had cut out a sloped chunk of cushion from inside the vinyl coated seat so he could stand flat-footed astride the bike. But now the seat wedges me forward so that my balls press against the gas tank, begging for mercy. When I get home, limping to the door, I wonder if I've made such a good choice after all.

Persistence, though, has a way of paying off. I remove and disassemble the carburetors again and clean them more thoroughly this time using an assortment of wire brushes. Then I change the oil and spark plugs and hire a local mechanic to adjust the valves and mount new tires. I get the mechanic to inspect the bike thoroughly, after which he says, "She's in perfect running condition."

Not long afterward, a dual bucket seat I ordered from the JC Whitney catalogue arrives, and it's like a pillow from heaven compared to that old seat. Then my father surprises me with a package from Florida in which there's a black leather

bomber's jacket he bought from Banana Republic. It fits as if
tailor-made. With renewed pride, I give the motorcycle a comprehen-
sive cleaning. I wash it and Armor All the seat, the backrest
and the new tires. I wax the tank and fairing, then polish the
chrome parts until they dazzle in the sunlight. After I'm done,
I stare at the bike for a long time, scrutinizing every inch, and
I can hardly look away. It's beautiful. I know the first place I
have to go. I have to show it off to Mr. John Doyle.

The motorcycle opens up a new world. Whereas before I
pretty much stayed within the confines of Terre Haute, now
I'm a regional explorer, going to all the little places of interest
I see on the map. There are covered bridges in Parke County
and an Amish settlement in East-Central Illinois. There are
peaceful state parks and lakes and quaint middle-class towns.
Pretty college campuses are also scattered throughout the re-
gion, all within an easy day's ride. Best of all is Bloomington,
Indiana, which has a university campus almost as lovely as
Auburn's and a vast improvement over the ugliness of ISU.

Indiana University offers two places of refuge—the library
and the student union—both of which are better than Auburn's
and light years superior to Indiana State's. I'm drawn to these
places like an insect to a street lamp. Any decent size project
that has to get done, I do in Bloomington, where my thinking
is sharper and my motivation equal to the task.

If it's warm enough, I ride the motorcycle through the two
lane country roads to get there. It takes about an hour. After
tooling around town, I park the bike at the library, and from
here the pattern is generally the same. With backpack in hand,
I go to the basement cafeteria where I buy coffee and a muffin.
I begin with a good book, like something by Herman Hesse, to
keep the positive energy flowing. The combined effect of coffee, sugary sweets, atmosphere and a good book is enough to

fire up the synapses for whatever else is needed.

After an hour or so of reading, I'm ready for the strain of my assigned work. This may last three or four hours, but the reward afterward is great. With the sense of freedom that comes from finishing work, I rummage around the stacks of this mammoth beast of a library, exploring deep into the night. Some nights it's the architecture or the literature shelves that draw me in. Sometimes it's quantum physics or the craft of writing or Eastern theology. Here I learn about the ways of meditation. And it's here that I begin to think about my curse in a new light. Through the wisdom found in these books, I can see beyond the delusion of crazy versus non-crazy and into the realm of being, learning what it might be like to be happy with myself. The good feeling lasts through the night.

Riding back to Terre Haute at two o'clock in the morning, I sometimes experience for a brief moment a thing I call motorcycle meditation. It's a kind of union with the bike that goes beyond just sitting on it and riding. It's as if the right hand and the throttle merge into one, as does the left hand with the clutch. The left foot shifts the gears, but the mechanics of ankle, foot and gearbox play together in common function. Right foot and right hand control the braking system, but again it's like an unconscious connection of body and brakes. Distinctions of foot, brake, hand and clutch are gone for the moment. Now bike-man has entered the realm of timelessness. The body is still, except for the critical movements controlling the bike. And the breath may well be coming in through the carburetor barrels and out through the exhaust. The wind, the street, the trees and the houses are all part of the mind's interior.

It's too bad when a stray thought comes in to mess the whole thing up, severing this spirit of unity, putting bike-man back into the realm of mundane reality.

33

L ATE in the summer of 1992, one of the secretaries in
the clinic tells me I haven't been paying as much attention as I should to the dress code. They want me
to dress like a professional, which means that I ought to be
wearing a tie, an ironed dress shirt and *absolutely no jeans.* I
don't like it and I wonder who did the complaining, but it's not
worth fighting over. I could tell the clinical director that a tie
is like a noose that separates a man's head from his heart, but
I don't think that'll help my cause.

Next morning I gather up a bunch of wrinkled shirts and
set up the ironing board by the TV in the living room. I'm not
much for ironing. It's a slow and frustrating task, and I'm not
good at it. It's also rare for me to be watching TV in the morning, and it's the first time in years that I happen upon the *Phil
Donahue Show.* It serves as background noise to numb out the
frustration of ironing.

Soon I find myself caught up in the program. On this particular show, Phil has on a bunch of men from an organization
called New Warrior, and they seem different from the men I

normally encounter. Instead of talking about the standard things men discuss, they're talking about their feelings and their true desires, and they're having fun doing it for Christ's sake. Another thing that attracts me is the calm resonance in their voices, making them sound strong and self-assured. I wonder what kind of strange brew they've been drinking. Whatever it is, I want it. When the show is over, I call the New Warrior number to have them send me a brochure. The guy on the phone gets my address and also mentions the Indiana Men's Council, which meets every month in Indianapolis. He says it's a good place to find guys who've gone through the New Warrior training. He gives me the address of a suburban church they use for their meetings.

With a chest full of fear I make the 70-mile drive east to Indianapolis, and I find the church the guy was talking about. The parking lot is filled with cars, which makes me think I'm late. It's reassuring to see others pull up behind me. Some of the men are carrying drums. Up ahead there's a group of men by the door exchanging hugs, and I'm afraid they'll be hugging me when I arrive. I can't help wondering whether I've dropped in on a gay pride encampment.

Meanwhile, there's a loud raucous sound coming from the church. Inside, I'm immersed in an unfamiliar earthy smell, later identified as burning sage, and I see men drumming with reckless abandon. Those without drums are dancing around in a circle, yelling or singing. It looks like high theatrics, like they're all drama queens. There must be 70 or 80 men in here, mostly white guys. I watch the fanfare as an outsider, feeling awkward as hell. I'm the only one not moving or drumming to the beat.

This activity goes on for a while until, finally, one of the older men stands in the center of the room with a decorative stick raised over his head. Momentarily the sound and frenetic activity rises to a yelling, banging chaos. Then the man in the center drives the stick down until it hits the floor and immediately the room goes silent.

We form into a large circle standing and holding hands. Then one of the leaders calls forth the spirits of our ancestors. He invites the seven directions to join our meeting—north, south, east, west, above, below and within—and he welcomes the powers associated with each direction to be present here tonight. I go through the motions, turning and facing the appropriate direction when we get to it. Next is a check-in process, which means that each man gets an opportunity to step into the circle, state his name and report what he's feeling at the moment.

I don't want to announce to the group that I'm scared as hell, but then I hear other men say that they're scared too, and they don't combust into flames after they've said it. So I figure it'll be okay. When it's my turn I say, "My name is Brett, and I'm feeling fear."

Later in the evening, there's a kind of open forum where any man can step into the middle of the circle and state his truth, whatever that is. It may be an issue he has with the group or with himself, or it may be something new in his life he wants to announce. There's no way I'm going in there. Armies would have to drag me in.

Other men are quick to approach the center where they stand, one after another, holding what they call the talking stick. One guy tells about his divorce and the shame he feels over failing to make it a better marriage. Another speaks of his struggle raising a teenage son and how hard it is to get close to the kid, despite his efforts. A couple of men talk about their meaningless jobs and how they wish they could quit.

There's one guy in the group who says he feels betrayed by another man in the circle, and he wants to clear up the matter. The alleged betrayer agrees to get in there. So the two men stand facing each other, both holding onto the stick. The guy who feels betrayed states his beef in a simple and direct way without waffling back and forth. The other guy acknowledges what he did and proposes a way to "get back into integrity" with this man he calls his friend. They work it out in an unflinching manner, and they both look thrilled to have the issue resolved. They mark the occasion with a hug.

Now I get a sense of what the hugging is about. It looks like support and honoring, rather than a queer thing. This place seems far removed from the cutthroat world of male competition. Still, I'm a skeptic.

It's strange though when I realize that the terrible fear I had when the meeting started is gone now. I feel relaxed, and there's even a little joy creeping in. Something good is happening here.

I decide to return to the next monthly gathering in Indianapolis and, in the fall of '92, I'll go through the New Warrior initiation weekend. It's supposed to be a kind of boot camp for a man's soul. I'll see what it does for mine.

To describe the events of the weekend would be to do injustice to the experience, and it's not allowed by the organization. Rightly so, they want new men to arrive without a lot of preconceived ideas about what will happen next. Without giving anything away, the weekend is partly a hard-edged confrontation, guided by rules of personal responsibility, and partly a rapid-fire journey for men to find their way in the world. It's like an invitation to open up your guts, look inside, see the good and the bad and then decide how you'll conduct yourself from here into the future. To me, the weekend is filled with a kind of unfamiliar brilliance.

As the weekend progresses, I get something I don't expect, which is a new sense of hopefulness about the world and myself in it. The leaders of the retreat have a way of pulling stuff out of me that I didn't know was in there. When they pry into the well of emotion below the surface, they don't run away, nor do they ask for restraints and syringes. Instead, they stand in front of me, look me in the eyes and guide me through the rage and the grief. When it's all over, I can feel some of the burdens I've been carrying for so many years melt away.

A few days after the initiation, there's a graduation ceremony, followed by weekly groups that carry on the spirit of the weekend. At the ceremony, when the hoopla is over, I work up the nerve to approach one of the older leaders and talk to him in private. I start by telling him how much I respect him for what he did during the weekend, then I ask him if he would meet with me from time to time.

It's not analysis or therapy I want. What I want, and maybe what I need, is mentoring from a wise elder who knows about the soul and how to tend to it. I know I won't find that in the ISU psychology department because *soul* is not a construct they're familiar with. It can't be plugged into a treatment protocol and therefore isn't relevant for teaching. But I think this wise old man has a pipeline to the soul. I can learn from him.

He agrees to my request, and we begin to have weekly meetings. His name is Don Jones. He's a former minister turned psychotherapist turned men's movement guru, and he's not the kind of man you can easily ignore. For one, he's tall and mighty looking with wiry white hair and eyes like an eagle's. But his voice is the thing that grabs you. I don't think there are rooms big enough to contain it. There's this resonance about it that comes from deep within the belly. You can't help but listen, especially when he's outdoors reciting a poem in full voice. I imagine the trees are vibrating then.

I get inspired anew each time I'm with Don, even when we're only eating burgers and fries at Hardee's, talking about normal everyday stuff. He has a way of taking a topic, almost any topic, and shedding a light of truth on it. Sometimes his observations are deep, which force me to contort my brain to understand them, and sometimes they're flat out hilarious. You can't help but laugh with him, even if he's laughing at himself. He knows how to be a purposeful jokester.

The best thing about being with him is the way he treats me as an equal, even though I know I'm not. It's as if he sees some kind of potential in me, and this is the person he's talking to, not the anxious graduate student that I embody everyday.

In my talks with Don, I get a kind of blessing that I've been waiting for. He tells me that my breakdown in 1984 was a spiritual crisis, as well as a spiritual wake-up call, and it's my job to see it as such. He says it's up to me to harness its potential. Then he says, "You're a big man playing small."

The statement pierces through me when he says it. It's a blessing and a criticism and a challenge, all at the same time, and it makes the hair at the back of my head stand on end. Maybe he's telling the story of my life in a few simple words.

Back in Terre Haute I continue to find diversions from the one-dimensionality of the psychology program. Fresh from the New Warrior weekend, I get together with Annette to run a therapy group at the Federal Penitentiary. We recruit about 10 male inmates, mostly drug offenders, to join the weekly group.

It's a tough road getting the men to talk about their troubled lives in the midst of their distrust. I know what that's like, and I realize I don't trust them either. Saying this aloud actually helps because it's the truth, and I think people respond better to the truth than to pre-packaged lies. At least that's normally the way it is.

Here in the prison group, there's a new level of truth telling and it seems liberating to some. A couple of the men can't handle it and quit the group, but others say it's the highlight of their week. Of course, the rest of their week isn't exactly a picnic. But I take it as a compliment just the same.

Annette and I muddle through the group for about two months, and we both find satisfaction in the progress we're making. But then we hear about some bureaucratic snafu. New regulations say we can't continue. What are these new regulations? The administrators won't say. Who made up the new regulations? They won't say. To find out the whole story and try to change the outcome is an exercise in futility. We drop it and move on to other pursuits. Meanwhile, we've left these men with their wounds open wide. Who cares about that?

34

I N the fall of '92 I take on another challenge. I decide to become a big brother, with the Big Brother Big Sister organization. I want to see what it would be like to be a father figure without the weighty responsibility of actually being a father. I'm also hoping to have a little buddy to take along with me on motorcycle treks around the region. I imagine it'll be fun traveling around with a kid, especially a kid who'll see these places for the first time. I wish I could see the world again with that kind of freshness.

First I have to go through the laborious process of becoming a big brother, which includes the paperwork, the interview, a background check, letters of recommendation and a home visit. As usual, I deny my psychiatric history, assuming there's no way they'll discover it on their own. My assumption is correct. After the process is over, I get to choose the kind of kid I want to spend time with. There are dozens of fatherless boys on the waiting list who never get chosen. It's a sad fact.

The boy I get is a seven-year-old, bi-racial kid named Anthony whose mother is white and whose long absent father is black. He's a smart and cheerful boy who no doubt loves his mother, but he's timid around men and doesn't get along with his stepfather. When I visit him for the first time (in the cruddy little trailer his family calls home) I can hardly get a word out of him. But there's a magic word for kids the world over at moments such as this—a word that has the effect of major transformation. I suggest we go to "McDonald's," and Anthony brightens up. Adding the words "Happy Meal" completes his transformation. From here on things will be okay.

The deal is that I meet Anthony every week for at least two hours, but it usually turns into four hours and sometimes more, depending on my schedule. In winter, we trudge around the mall and play mindless video games. We go to the mall's bookstore or the local library and bury ourselves in books, and then we talk about what we've read. We rent the *Star Wars* trilogy and spread it out over three visits.

On a snow covered day in late February we find perhaps the only hill in Terre Haute to go sledding on borrowed sleds. It's the first time sledding for both of us, and it's terrific fun. There's a bonfire burning on top of the hill where people are gathered with hot chocolate. A little girl is selling cups of it for 75 cents, but we're too busy sledding to bother. We trade off sleds with other kids to see which ones are fastest, and we cheer the kid who makes it all the way down without flipping.

Driving home, I turn on the radio to catch the day's news. In Lower Manhattan part of the World Trade Center was just bombed. An unknown number of people are either dead or wounded.

The spirit of the day has changed. I tell Anthony about a thing called terrorism. I say these people have lost touch with their hearts, which means they can do anything without regard for others. We talk about how scary that is. "Never lose sight of what's in your heart," I say. It's good advice for both of us.

❈

With springtime approaching I mention the motorcycle to Anthony's mother and ask whether he could go for rides with me. I tell her I'll buy him a quality helmet and drive with extra caution. I can tell she's frightened at the thought of it and wants to say no, but the words "all right" come out of her mouth instead. Once Anthony discovers what she said, there'll be no chance for her to take it back.

So in the spring of '93 my travels with Anthony begin. First we ride around the streets of Terre Haute to get him over his initial fear. Then we take a short trip to Parke County with its timeless farms and red covered bridges, some of which are still open to traffic. In the tiny village of Bridgeton, we pull over at a pig farm and make snorting noises at the pigs. Then we ride to Rockville, the county seat, where we order slices of pie at a little café.

I don't realize it on our first trip, but later I discover that Rockville is known as a hotbed of Ku Klux Klan activity. It's true that when I look around town I don't see any black people here, and the cars are all American made. The town is as white-bread conservative as a town gets, reminding me of sitcoms from the 1950's. The police station, which is a few doors down from the café, looks like it popped out of *The Andy Griffith Show*. And yet, despite my vigilance for the goddamn racists, the town feels warm and inviting. It's a world apart from Anthony's trailer park and the rundown neighborhood surrounding it.

In the span of a couple of months, Anthony and I have traveled to a good many desirable spots in the region, like Bloomington and Nashville, Indiana. We've stopped in Greencastle and Crawfordsville and the Shades State Park, none of which Anthony had ever seen before. To give him greater decision-making power over where we go I take out the map and, using a compass, make a circle around Terre Haute with a 60-mile radius. Then I have him pick a town on or near the circle, to a place we haven't been to yet. That's where we go, unless I override him with my veto power. We saddle up with maps, water bottles and M&M's for Anthony to snack on if the scenery gets boring.

On one of our early trips we cross the Wabash River and head into Illinois. I park the bike at the state line. There we stand side-by-side, him in Illinois and me in Indiana. Then we switch states and shake hands across the imaginary line, as if we're important dignitaries acknowledging each state's right to exist. For Anthony there's a new awareness developing. He begins to realize there's not a damn bit of difference between Western Indiana and Eastern Illinois.

With this exercise in triviality complete, we go on to find the Amish community in East-Central Illinois, near Arcola. I tell Anthony that you can spot which homes are Amish because there are no power or phone lines going from the road to the houses. So he looks for these indicators and taps me whenever he finds an example. "Look, another Amish house," he says.

Soon we're deep into Amish country on two lane roads where there aren't any power lines at all. I notice the names on the mailboxes, many of which are the same, and I can't help wondering about genetic inbreeding. When I see a plain-looking woman with droopy brows, my suspicion deepens. They could use a stud service here, I'm thinking, but I try not to dwell on it, and I don't tell Anthony what's in my deviant brain.

At times we ride behind a horse and buggy, and I can tell Anthony is all excited about it. "Look, look!" he yells while patting me on the back.

We stop along the side of the road on a dirt shoulder to watch Amish farmers tending their fields. They're working the ground with a horse drawn cultivator, and they can see us watching. We wave to be polite. I figure this is a good spot to rest a bit. I stretch and grab a water bottle for Anthony and me, and I take out a couple of granola bars.

While checking the oil, I see a man and a young girl walking toward us. I put the dipstick back and say "Hello." The man greets us back and then gives me a compliment on the motorcycle.

"Thanks," I say and proceed to give him a compliment on the beauty of the property. I want to keep the conversation going because I figure this could be a good civics lesson for Anthony, maybe better than he'll get in his social studies class.

I introduce Anthony and myself to the farmer, and he does the same, telling us the girl is his daughter. She doesn't say a word the whole time but hardly ever takes her eyes off us. I can't imagine the kinds of thoughts she's having. Thankfully, she doesn't have the droopy brow syndrome.

I tell the man about a conversation I had with Anthony, in which I explained that Amish people don't have any televisions in their homes and how shocked Anthony was at this bit of news.

The farmer laughs a little and says to Anthony, "Yes that's right. We've seen televisions in stores, but we don't have any at home." He goes on to tell us about the kinds of things he and his family do instead of watching TV. The list is long, and it's told with gentleness, as if the boundaries of age, culture and race are easy things to overcome.

While the man is talking, I can see that Anthony is taking it in, and I'm hoping it'll leave an impression. Like most kids, he's wedded to the television as if it's another bodily appendage, lured by messages of instant gratification. I'd like to see Anthony live here in this man's home for a month and see what it does for him. It's too bad such a thing isn't possible.

When the conversation is over, I thank the man and wish him well. I think he's given Anthony something of value today and I hope it sticks. I want to return the favor and say something wise for his little girl to hold onto, but there's nothing

I can come up with. I think she sees Anthony and me as a couple of dopey outsiders who've lost their way on a flashy machine.

Anthony and I get back on the bike and ride off, waving goodbye to our new acquaintances. In the solitude of the community the motorcycle is loud, and I think of how obnoxious it must sound. It's far too loud for this place. It takes a few miles for it to sound right again.

On the phone I tell my mother that Anthony doesn't have a bicycle, nor does he know how to ride one. "Every kid should have a bike," my mother says.

"I know but there's nothing I can do about it right now." It's like fishing with a baited hook, and I half know what's coming next.

In a few days a check arrives from my mother for the purpose of buying Anthony a bike. I go to the local Wal-Mart and pick out a black one that looks kind of like a motorcycle. In my living room I assemble the thing, and when complete I hide it under a thick brown blanket.

I go to pick up Anthony without telling him about the new bike. Instead, I act all suspicious while opening the back door of my house. It looks like someone's broken in, I tell him, because I swear the door was locked when I left. In the kitchen, walking toward the living room, I pull Anthony aside and give him the "Shhh" sign. Shaking with feigned nerves, I whisper, "Look over there. I think it's a robber hiding under the blanket."

Anthony looks sufficiently scared.

Then I reach into the closet for weaponry suitable for the task of knocking out robbers. I take the mop and give Anthony the broom. Walking on tiptoes, I lead the way to the brown mound with my mop poised for attack. Before we get there, Anthony tugs at my shirt and whispers in my ear, "Maybe we should call the police."

"Yeah, we will, but first we gotta make sure he can't get away."

Then, when it looks like Anthony's too scared and ready to bolt or urinate in his pants, I grab the blanket and pull it back, revealing the shiny new bike.

"Look, it's a new bike just for you."

He smiles and jumps toward the thing like a dazed rabbit. Then we walk it over to Collette Park where, for the next two hours, I teach Anthony how to ride a bike.

By sunset, after about a dozen falls, he's learned how to handle it pretty well. He wants to keep riding after dark and doesn't care about eating dinner or going home after that. I have to get tough with him and order him to walk the bike back to the house. He does so, sulking the whole way. I remind him to be grateful for the gift, sent from a secret admirer down in Florida, and I remind him of the day's accomplishment. "Learning to ride a bike—that's big stuff," I tell him, "especially without training wheels."

His sulking winds down, and I can see the look of pride surfacing on his face.

35

To live in the Midwest cut off from the world of farming is to miss the better part of living in the Midwest. I'm lucky to have a farming connection, which is surprisingly due to my father. Down in Fort Lauderdale, my dad leases the office next to his to a lawyer named Joanne. They become friends, and soon my father learns that her parents have a farm near Terre Haute, next to the miniscule town of Brazil.

I meet Joanne's parents during winter break in Florida, and they tell me I should come by and visit them at their farm sometime. I say I will, only half expecting to do so, but I get reminders from my dad and Joanne, which make it almost impossible not to visit.

My first trip to the farm of Jack and Jan Hoffman is by way of motorcycle. Riding down the white gravel driveway, I see a three-legged dog making a feeble effort to chase after me. Jan comes out to meet me, telling me the dog's name is Pokey. She says Jack found the dog left for dead after a hunter shot him. Rather than let the poor thing die, he rushed him to a vet-

erinarian and then adopted him—minus a hind leg—naming
him Pokey. The big brown mutt has the run of the place, but he
mostly stays close to the main barn where he's got everything
a three-legged dog could want. He's about the most contented
dog I've ever seen.

After Pokey, it's my motorcycle that draws attention. Jack
looks her over and says, "She's a pretty machine." He asks
how she rides and about the engine. I can tell he's actually interested in knowing the answers. Then he focuses on the chain
and says, "You know that looks like it could use a cleaning."

I tell him I've been a little neglectful about that, which
feels like confessing a great sin. I can see that his farm is immaculate. The tractors and the combine shine as if freshly
waxed, and all the tools in the barn are dust free and in their
proper places. I've never seen a workplace so well maintained,
and I'm a little awestruck by it. The effect of it increases the
guilt I feel over my grimy motorcycle chain.

But Jack has the answer to my woes. He gets out a couple
of old toothbrushes and a de-greasing agent made especially
for O-ring chains. Then he gets down in a baseball catcher's
position and works the bristles through the links of the chain. I
watch him cleaning a good part of it like a pro while I'm standing off to the side like a statue, feeling guilty again.

"Here, I'll take over," I say. I put the bike on its center-stand
and scrub the chain, trying to do exactly as Jack demonstrated,
since there's no improving upon perfection. Meanwhile, Jack
goes back to the barn to get a variety of other cleaning products so we can make the whole bike shine.

Soon the spirit of cleaning takes over and it leads to renewed pride. I feel like the wayward son who sinned but has
now found his way back to redemption. With my newly immaculate motorcycle, I'm in harmony with the workings of
the farm.

Here on the Hoffman farm, things work exactly as they

should. Nothing is broken. Nothing is neglected. If a thing exists here, it exists with purpose. Why should it be any other way? Why possess a thing that diminishes your pride and wears away at your sense of wholeness? Being on this farm is to approach that feeling of wholeness again.

While giving me a tour of the property, Jack talks about the yearly cycle of corn farming and the equipment required for each step of the process. He shows me the silos where the grain is kept, and he talks about the different machines. It seems the older the machine is, the more favor Jack shows when describing its function.

And he values the simple just as much as the complex. Jack takes out an old scythe and shows me how to use it properly. He's a thin man of about 70 with a broad smile, and he stands up straight, the way a man is supposed to stand. Working with the scythe, he clears a swath of grass as if it's an art form, like something out of a Tai Chi demonstration. Then he hands me the tool so I can give it a go.

It's an awkward strain when I first try it. I'm bending the wrong way, which strains my back, and I can't get an even cut. Jack patiently tells me what I'm doing wrong, directing me to the proper adjustments, and before long I'm sweeping down tufts of grass with precision. After a few minutes I ask Jack why people don't use scythes anymore to cut grass.

"Well, I guess people have forgotten how to use it," he says, "and they're just being lazy."

One of Jack's newest acquisitions is the behemoth combine—the top of the line—featuring an enclosed air-conditioned cabin equipped with contoured seats and a fine stereo system. Sitting in the driver's seat, surveying the switches and gauges galore, it feels like I'm sitting in the cockpit of an airline jet. It's that powerful feeling of sitting high above the common folk, controlling a powerful machine.

While climbing down from the combine, I notice something that doesn't fit the surroundings. It's a wasp's nest attached to the frame of the garage opening, and there are wasps buzzing around it. I ask Jack why he hasn't knocked the thing down.

His response surprises me. He says with a broad smile, "The wasps have just as much right to the place as we do."

Then his wife Jan tells me a story that has to be among the most unusual accounts I've ever heard. She says there are times when a wasp unwittingly flies into the cabin of the combine and ends up spending the day out in the field with Jack.

I'm thinking that wasp wouldn't last more than five minutes in there with me. If he doesn't sting me first I'd squash his guts, first chance I get.

But Jack's reverence for the living creatures of the world is far greater than mine. Instead of squashing the bug, Jan tells how Jack rides with the wasp all day long, never getting annoyed or stung. If for some reason he has to stop the combine and get out to check something, he makes sure the wasp stays in the cabin. If the wasp gets too anxious and flies out through the door, Jack shoos him back into the cabin and shuts the door.

Shocked, I ask, "Why the hell would you do a thing like that?"

He says it's because the wasp would never be able to find its way back to the nest. "I don't want the poor fella suffering out there in the cornfield," he says with a wide smile.

I look over at Jan in disbelief, wondering if they're playing a joke on me, but they're not. "You've got some kind of husband there," I say to Jan.

She smiles at Jack, and he smiles back at her.

When I get to know Jack and Jan better, I realize they have a kind of ideal relationship. They're kind and loving toward each other, and it isn't the sappy kind of love you see in Hollywood movies. I can also tell how much they respect each other's opinion. Whenever they work on something together, they have fun doing it, and it shows in the quality results they get. Their farm is cleaner and more orderly than the ones nearby. When the growing season reaches its climax, the Hoffman corn is taller with a deeper shade of green than the adjacent cornfields. Maybe their relationship and their optimism help the crop grow as well as it does.

The thing I want to know is how to find a match like the one I see in Jack and Jan Hoffman. I know what a rarity such a thing is, but I figure it's still worth a shot. First, I want to know how they met. They tell me about a community dance in the little village of Clinton, Indiana. I guess all towns of a certain size had these dances back then, and the ones in Clinton were no different from countless others. There was a disc jockey spinning popular records of the big bands, and there were starry-eyed adolescents trading dance partners and drinking punch between dances. It sounds like a great way to make that love connection.

The way Jack and Jan tell it, they fell in love right away, but maybe it took them both awhile to realize it. No matter, it's been love ever since. They make it seem like the most effortless thing in the world. It just flows.

I tell them about the troubles with dating nowadays and how I'm meeting all the wrong women. It's gotten to the point where I've stopped looking. The ideal woman would have to drop out of the sky from a dirigible and land on my car the way things are going. But Jack and Jan keep saying optimistic things like, "be patient" and "she's around" and "it'll happen." When it doesn't happen right away, I feel like I'm letting them down, bursting their optimistic bubble.

By October the Hoffmans are busy harvesting their corn. In mid-November the daylight is diminishing and it's too cold to ride the motorcycle. I put her away for the winter, knowing she'll be ready again next April.

My weekly visits with Anthony now include trips to the Hoffman farm. A highlight for Anthony is to play around with Pokey in a game of chase, which is a close contest given the dog's physical handicap. For me, the highlights are the conversation and the hearty meal. It's the closest thing to having a family in Indiana. After dessert and tea, the drive home in the blackness of the rural night sky is a time of sadness.

As winter sets in, I realize Anthony doesn't have a pair of gloves. So I give him a pair, telling him to keep them together in a place he'll remember.

By the next week he can't find them, and I'm stuck waiting in Anthony's cluttered mess of a trailer while he rummages through piles of dirty laundry. After all the searching he still can't find them. So we go to Wal-Mart to get him new gloves. I keep my mouth shut about not losing this pair because I think he's learned his lesson, but I'm still afraid they'll disappear like the others.

A couple of weeks later, my fear is realized when he's lost this newest pair of gloves. I give him some gym socks to wear on his hands while we're outdoors. Within a few days my mother comes to the rescue again by sending up another pair of gloves—a far better pair than the ones I got him. As I place them in his hands I tell him, "These are really good gloves, the kind you definitely don't want to lose."

I take Anthony, fresh gloves and all, to Deming Park for some ice-skating on the frozen pond. I'm told they don't have any skates large enough to fit me, but Anthony gets a pair that fits fine. He's never ice-skated before, and I've done it only once at a rink in Miami in the late 1970's. That was with Phil and his sister, and I remember failing miserably at it. Still I figure I should be able to teach Anthony, as long as he thinks I know what I'm talking about.

Anthony starts with his feet spread out like a duck's, and sure enough he falls ass-backward. I pull him up, preaching the virtues of keeping your feet parallel. He doesn't know what the word means yet, so I tell him about railroad tracks and how he should focus on keeping his feet that way. "Railroad tracks," I say every time he falls. I'm like a broken record.

In a little while, by God, he gets it. I feel like a proud father watching him zoom around the pond. When he comes back after the final run, I tell him how proud I am of his improvement. "When you first started you really stunk up the pond, but now you're skating great."

As he's untying the laces on his skates, I notice a TV news reporter interviewing a bunch of kids near Anthony. After a couple of quick interviews, she comes over to him and asks about the skating. This is considered newsworthy reporting in Terre Haute. Anthony looks up at the camera with the microphone poised near his mouth and says, "I really stunk up the pond when I first started, but then I got to skating great." His was one of the few interviews to make it on the evening news.

A week after our shining moment in the Terre Haute spotlight, Anthony and I drive around town, running errands before dinner, stopping at the all important Wal-Mart. On the drive home I notice Anthony is wearing only one glove. I pull the car over and ask him about the missing glove. He says he thinks he might've left it in the parking lot.

By this time my patience for missing gloves is running thin, and I don't understand this business of leaving personal belongings in parking lots. Anthony tries to explain it, but I can't bear another excuse. I think it's time for a more pointed demonstration.

I remove the black leather gloves from my hands. Then I say to him, "Anthony, look at these gloves. Look closely. See the initials right there? Those are my initials, written by my mother. She bought me these gloves before I went off to college in 1983." I pause for effect. "That's two years before you were born! And I still have them."

The point of my little lecture is to invoke the proper balance of shame and respect. Respect for things kept and valued and not lost. I don't know if it works, but it makes me feel better. Afterward, we drive back to Wal-Mart to scour the goddamn parking lot.

36

W ITH the arrival of spring '94, my thoughts turn to leaving Terre Haute and to the future beyond. The last part of the doctoral program is a yearlong internship, which involves the practice and study of psychology in a professional setting alongside other psychologists. The internship I've chosen is in Albany, New York, which is where I'll be heading in late July.

One reason for choosing Albany is that I want to return to the Northeast, not too far from Philadelphia or Boston. By now my sister Julia, who also graduated from Auburn, lives in Boston on Commonwealth Avenue with her husband and their two dogs. In Philadelphia, there's my aunt and uncle and cousin, who give me the red carpet treatment whenever I visit. I've also got a couple of friends from Villanova I like to see. Albany is a great location to launch these sorts of weekend road trips.

And there's another reason for settling in Albany. Two professors at Indiana State, a husband and wife, defected from the Midwest to teach at a college near Albany. They were my favorite professors, and now they've become good friends. Starting a new life with them nearby will do me a world of good.

In early July I gear up for the next big move. All of my classes are finished, and I've successfully defended my doctoral project. That meeting went over as smooth as silk. There were no tough questions I couldn't handle and no major changes called for. It's as good as done. I've jumped over all the hurdles at ISU with hardly a snag, and now they're letting me go with their blessing for a bright future. All that remains is my internship and then the state license exam. These are two manageable steps, after which I'll be a psychologist. They're actually going to make me a psychologist.

The question remaining in the back of my brain is whether or not I really want to be a psychologist. For now, I'm too busy getting my degree to mull that over. For better or worse I'm on a mission, and I won't let a question like that get in the way.

My friends Carl and Jeff have agreed to help me with a yard sale. I put an ad in the local paper, stating that it begins at nine o'clock in the morning. But apparently yard sale buyers are as eager as they get here in Terre Haute. By 7:30 I've got people browsing around the place while I'm still trying to price stuff, and Carl and Jeff won't be here for another hour.

The first thing I sell is an old futon, then an electric range that isn't even mine. The old house I've been living in has all kinds of junk in the basement from previous renters, mostly former graduate students. Since no one else can claim the stuff, I consider it an inheritance. This means I'm selling stuff I hardly recognize, acting like it's dear to my heart. It's a good day's gig.

Finally my friends show up. Jeff puts out a row of African drums he's trying to sell, and when there's a lull in the flow of buyers I bring out my motorcycle as a decoy to draw in more customers. *I see you like the motorcycle, but wouldn't you rather take home this lovely record player?* It's the old bait-and-switch strategy, and it actually works.

As the day rolls on I sell a washing machine and a dryer, a dog kennel, a small TV, an old computer, a lawn mower, throw rugs, clothes, books and a window air conditioner. I even manage to sell the record player and some old records for a total of eight dollars. By late afternoon, I get a little carried away when I sell the drafting table that I built with my father back in 1986.

We built the table after I made the decision to major in industrial design at Auburn. It has aluminum legs fixed onto an oak frame, and the top is marine plywood with a Formica surface. The whole thing came from scraps out of my dad's garage, but the final effect is pure originality and function. The top is a split-level design, with the main portion adjusting to a near vertical position, while the smaller right side portion remains stationary. That's the place to put your coffee and your drawing instruments.

The woman who wants it offers the asking price of $35, saying it'll be perfect for the kind of work she does. I want to take it back and tell her I've changed my mind, but there'll be no place in my new apartment to put it. It's hard to look as she loads the table onto her truck, just like it was hard letting go of my old El Camino. Someday I'll build another table just like that one, except for the aluminum legs.

My mood brightens when I count up all the profits from the sale. The total is just under $900, which is far more than I expected. Thank you Terre Haute! With this money I can pay for the moving truck. Plus, I have a certain airline ticket I needed to buy, and now I can.

A few weeks before the yard sale, I called Phil to ask if he would ride with me from Terre Haute to Albany and help me unload the truck into my new apartment. He agreed, as long as

I pay for his plane ticket.

All the goodbyes are tough to handle. There's Don Jones, Jack and Jan Hoffman, and my professors and friends from the program. Then there's Anthony—my toughest goodbye of all. I know we'll see each other again and talk on the phone, but it won't be the same. I want him to know that I've enjoyed every minute with him, even the tough times, and I want him to know that I'm proud of him. I want him to realize he's done as much for me as I have for him. In my head, I think it's important to tell him all these things.

But when I see him for the last time, all I can do is give him a hug, tell him I love him and cry. He cries and says he loves me too. And that's how we leave it.

The bigger tears come when I drive away from his squalid little trailer for the last time.

The next day Carl and Jeff arrive to help me load the moving truck—one with air conditioning this time. We load it without any trouble, which I could say is a testament to my vast furniture moving experience. It also doesn't hurt to have sold over half of my belongings in a yard sale.

The last piece to go on the truck is a little tricky. It's the motorcycle. With Carl and Jeff on either side, I drive it up the ramp and then fish her back and forth until she's near the left side. Carl straps her against the wall while I put cushions in between the wall and the bike. It seems tight, but with the momentum of the truck, she'll no doubt roll back and forth—all 600 pounds of her. We need to find a way to stop this.

Carl has the answer. Taking a couple of two-by-fours and nailing them to the floor of the truck, he wedges both tires in place. When he's done, I ask, "Do you think they'll notice the nail holes?"

"Not a chance," Carl says.

Soon I'm on the road heading east to the Indianapolis Airport. It's the moment I've thought about since I first arrived four years ago—seeing Terre Haute in my rearview mirror for the last time. It's a triumphant moment, but there's a feeling of loss in it too. For all its ugliness and flatness, I'll miss this town. Or, more accurately, I'll miss its people—Terre Hautian Hoosiers, Midwesterners to the core. You could say they're simple folks with a naïve sort of optimism. It's the kind of attitude that tells them to greet each new day as if the pain from the day before is gone forever. They seem to know there's no sense chasing after silly dreams. For them it's the day-to-day struggle that matters most. It may have something to do with geography. There's no coastline or mountains to fix upon and dream about. It's a flat existence, and it helps to endure it with pride.

I'm grateful to have learned alongside these people. It occurs to me that I didn't just come out here to get a degree in psychology. I came to experience life. While I've been here, I found a way to live it a little better. When I'm old and shriveled, these are the experiences I want to remember, more than just the doctoral degree.

When I get to the Indianapolis Airport I find that it's impossible to park the truck anywhere except the remote parking lot, half a mile from the main terminal. I don't care though. Walking is good, and I'm about 30 minutes early for Phil's flight anyway.

He's now married and living in a Virginia suburb just outside Washington, DC, where he works for a meat distribution company called Colorado Prime. He's learned the essence of quality meats, and if you ask him he'll tell you reams about the subject. Get him started on marbling or the quality difference between store-bought meats versus meats served in a high priced restaurant, and you'll be sorry.

When his plane arrives, Phil and I greet each other with

a hug and head out to the truck, talking nonstop. I show him the map and the route we'll be taking, telling him we should arrive in Albany by around nine o'clock tomorrow morning, allowing for pit stops along the way. In the high energy of the moment, I know the trip will be an effortless jaunt.

The sun sets behind us as we approach the highway.

As the miles go by Phil and I cover a wide range of subject matter and, with the help of a caffeine buzz, the conversation tends toward the ridiculous. We talk about societal trends, like the fact that everyone seems to be working longer, with a greater number of stores staying open 24 hours a day. Frantic commerce never seems to end, and it appears as though the demise of leisure time is imminent, despite technology's promise of giving us more free time. We wonder why people are working so hard anyway.

Then we come up with a proposal that the whole country must take a certain day off, like the first Friday of every month. No one would be allowed to work except for those employed by essential services, such as hospitals, police and fire departments. Otherwise—nothing—no TV stations broadcasting, no stores or gas stations operating and no transportation services. If you checked into a hotel on Thursday, you couldn't check out until Saturday.

We call it *Grounded Day*, and we think it's pretty brilliant—a genius idea concocted in the buzz of a long drive. For a while it seems like a real possibility. Citizens could lobby Congress, after which Congress would surely see the wisdom in it and pass the necessary legislation.

But then we let the idea slip into oblivion, along with all the other impossible dreams.

Around 3 A.M. we stop for a second or third cup of coffee and another in a series of late night snacks. We walk to the service plaza stiff from sitting so long, as if every appendage has turned prosthetic.

"We gotta loosen up, get the kinks out," I say.

Phil nods in agreement.

So we do what comes naturally. We take out a football and toss it back and forth under the light of the street lamps. After some stationary throws, we run patterns, congratulating each other when a pass is completed.

"Good throw."

"Good catch."

And "Shit" after dropping the ball when it was "right there in my hands!" No grandmothers are here to correct our language.

Back in the truck, we feel refreshed and ready for the next leg of the journey. With plenty of coffee and enough doughnuts to last until daybreak, we're a pair of happy travelers. And what do happy travelers do?

One thing they do is sing and, in our case, sing badly. We start with the goofy songs we listened to as kids, like *Billy Don't be a Hero* and *The Night Chicago Died* and *Benny and the Jets* and *Kodachrome*. Then we move on to our own compositions, like *The Black Dog Crapped on the Fence* and *I Love to Carry Fertilizer up the Hills of Montezuma*. Whether Montezuma has hills or not, we couldn't say. It's just a brainless lyric with a good flow.

We cap it off with our favorite little ditty, *Razor Blades*. We sing it in round style, like the way preschool kids sing *Row, Row, Row Your Boat*. It goes like this:

Razor blades, razor blades,
They are very sharp; they can cut you.
Razor blades, razor blades,
They are very sharp; they can cut you.
I don't know where you can buy them,
But Gillette makes the best.

After the singing, we pass some miles in silence. It's a good moment for both of us—to have come this far and still remain best friends. That has to count for something.

In the midst of our silence, it occurs to me that this curse I've carried for 10 years—this fear of going crazy—is fading out of my consciousness. I can feel it fading into nothing. All that remain are the lessons I've learned and the people who taught them.

High above the cabin of the truck, in the pale black sky, the Moon glows, just as it has for millions of years and just as it did in 1984. Nothing has changed since then. Yet everything is different. And that's fine with me.

The gallery of prophets will have to wait.

Epilogue

OVER two decades have passed since my psychotic episode, and throughout these years I've remained wary of the forces of psychiatry and the pharmaceutical industry. Despite so-called advancements in pharmacology, I wonder whether patients are any better off now than I was in 1984. Before exploring the issue further, a couple of caveats are in order. First, I believe there are good psychiatrists out there and even a few great ones who have spoken out against the overuse of medication. Second, I agree with those who say that some of these drugs are helpful for a small minority of patients, and I don't recommend flushing one's prescription drugs down the toilet as I did. Immediate withdrawal of neuroleptics can lead to a variety of problems, including an unnatural rebound back into psychosis. Thankfully, this never happened in my case.

The most compelling problem as I see it is the widespread practice of instantly drugging psychotic symptoms as soon as they emerge. This knee-jerk, reactive treatment has been in force since the 1950's and continues unchallenged. The basis for this approach is the biochemical-disease model of mental illness, which posits that patients have an imbalance of certain neurotransmitters in the brain. The assumption is that this alleged chemical imbalance is the *cause* of the patient's schizophrenia. But in fact this theory is based solely on correlational data. A significant cause and effect relationship has never been demonstrated. Further, the theory is equally plausible in reverse, meaning that it is just as valid to conclude that schizophrenia, itself, causes an imbalance. This alternative theory has not been given proper attention.

Meanwhile drug companies, backed by highly paid psychiatrists, promote the chemical imbalance theory as if proven truth. And, as a society, we accept it as truth because the term has been hammered into our heads for so long that it's become common knowledge and because we want to believe it. We want drugs that will cure whatever afflictions come our way, and we want them now. In this way, we are like a nation of adolescents, demanding instant fixes without further reflection. Drug companies are eager to satisfy our demands. They tout their newest medications as the best ones—sure to create a revolution in treatment—putting forth multi-million dollar campaigns to make their case. The hoopla is necessary for business because the older drugs have been turned over to the generic market and are thus no longer profitable. Free samples of the new drugs are initially offered to bait the doctor and the patient, and then, once baited, exorbitant prices are charged. Patients are typically encouraged to stay on the drugs for many years. This has become one of the most lucrative business practices in our post-industrial age.

In the midst of this madness it's important to remember one central fact, which is that drugs do not cure mental illness. Cure is a strong word, implying known cause and effect, as in the example of bacterial infection and antibiotic treatment. But even after all our scientific searching, we still know very little about the true causes of mental illnesses. Cure also requires that we define the diseased condition with precision. But most mental illnesses, including schizophrenia, cannot be diagnosed in such a manner. A quick look at the current version of psychiatry's diagnostic manual shows that there are five different types of schizophrenia with seven manifestations of each type. Additionally, there are the related diagnoses of schizoaffective disorder, schizophreniform disorder, brief reactive psychosis and six types of delusional disorders. This adds up to 43 supposedly distinct conditions!

The problem is that these 43 distinctions have become meaningless because all of these patients are treated the same. We haven't explored the very real possibility that different groupings might respond differently to drugs versus alternative treatment. Instead, we drug them all immediately as if they were all one bloc of mental disease. This is the essence of hammerhead medicine, as true now as it was in 1984.

The drugs used to treat schizophrenia have a wide variety of effects, only one of which may temporarily suppress psychotic symptoms. Meanwhile, even with the latest drugs, patients experience an array of adverse side effects. It's not farfetched to say that drug treatment of schizophrenia is similar to recommending alcohol for its beneficial effect on anxiety. Never mind the associated side effects of alcohol. By using the same logic of the drug companies and mainstream psychiatry, one could argue that anxiety is caused by a lack of alcohol and that alcohol is the treatment of choice for anxiety. This is foolish of course, but similar reasoning applies to schizophrenia and the neurotransmitter-blocking drugs.

Good logic suggests that these drugs may actually delay one's cure. In his exceptional book *Mad in America* (2002) Robert Whitaker revealed that less-developed countries like Nigeria, Columbia and India, which have little access to neuroleptic drugs, have far better treatment outcomes than those in developed countries, such as the United States. Moreover, despite so-called advancements in drug therapy, treatment outcomes for schizophrenics in the United States have actually *worsened* over the past hundred years. This suggests that long-term drug use is bad treatment. My view is that these drugs effectively keep patients locked in a semi-vegetative state where little productive processing can occur. Again, this is similar to the use of alcohol for the treatment of anxiety. The longer the person remains addicted to alcohol, the less likely he or she is to develop positive coping skills. The drug becomes the problem.

My advice to patients being treated for a psychotic condition is to be ever skeptical of psychiatric treatment and the highly touted effects of the drugs. Be wary of drug research as well because it is often funded by the drug manufacturer and is therefore prone to bias and deceptive reporting of results. Be aware that drug company influence goes well beyond doctors and medical journals and TV commercials. For example, the country's largest patient support group, National Alliance for the Mentally Ill, receives the bulk of its funding from the pharmaceutical industry and is almost uniformly pro-drugging. And finally, stay out of the hospital if you can. An inpatient stay almost guarantees that you will be treated with drugs, and your refusal to take them will not be looked upon with favor.

We are now entrenched in a dark age in which, from the top of the hierarchy, big business dictates the way we treat and conceptualize psychosis. Despite the obvious allure of money and quick fixes, when we reduce human experience down to neurotransmitters, we belittle ourselves and the patients we treat, and we close our minds to alternative approaches. For example, we have essentially stopped investigating the more abstract notion of inner conflict and how this may contribute to psychosis. And the notion of treating psychotic disorders without resorting to drugs is almost uniformly rejected. But, thankfully, this current state of affairs is not the final word. In time, we may enter into a new era—one that won't be dictated by drug money or the public's infatuation with the quick fix. At some critical point, I believe we will shift out of our current dark age and into a new light of understanding. Only then will patients get the mental health treatment they deserve.

More than a decade has passed since my departure from Terre Haute. In that time, I completed my internship and passed the license exam. I began my career as a psychologist by working with children and families in a rundown clinic in Schenectady, New York. After about 18 months of feeling powerless to change the lives of my clients, I shifted to the other extreme by working with elderly residents in three Upstate New York nursing homes. I did this for about four years, which was plenty of time for me to develop a new sense of powerlessness—namely, to the effects of aging and physical decline. Working with these residents made me feel as if my own aging process was accelerating.

Meanwhile, my bank account rose to the level where I could buy my first house in 1997. This marked the beginning of my immersion into the world of home improvement. Destroying the old and building the new became a new mission, and it took up the bulk of my free time. While restoring stability to the house, I also built a few pieces of furniture, including a new version of my old drafting table sold in the yard sale.

I shifted to my current job in 1999, working for a firm that conducts disability evaluations. The job requires me to travel across New York State and beyond to regional clinics, where I see the full spectrum of humanity. These are people applying for disability benefits or hoping to keep their current benefits from being cut off. In a way, it's like working in a hospital emergency room because you never know what kind of person you'll see from one moment to the next. A single day's work may include a brain injured truck driver, a depressed transsexual, a lead exposed child and a Vietnam combat veteran suffering from post-traumatic stress disorder. It's the kind of job that keeps me alert and as open-minded as I can be.

A few months after the tragedy of September 11, I met the woman who would later become my wife. Our first encounter occurred at a gym among the array of cardiovascular machines. With an impressive set of breasts and an equally impressive smile, she was beautiful. When the machine next to her opened up, I summoned the courage to get on it, and I introduced myself. She smiled and said her name was Sarah. We talked for a while and the conversation flowed smoothly, like we knew each other from some other time. It was surprisingly easy when I asked her out to lunch. She accepted and said she'd be happy to see me again. As she made her exit from the exercise room, she paused at the threshold of the door and looked back at me, smiling one last time. It felt like a smile from all the feminine energies of the universe. I knew at that moment that Sarah would become my wife.

Throughout the years that Sarah and I have been together, I've realized that I finally found what I was looking for. After all the searching, I can now say that we have the kind of rare love I saw between Jack and Jan Hoffman. It was worth the long wait. Maybe I needed all those years of being alone in order to be fully present in marriage. But I've always been a slow learner.

As life flows through its many changes, there's a constancy that remains, like a thread holding everything together. I think both the changes and the permanence are essential. While the cycle of change keeps life interesting, it's the sense of constancy that makes us feel whole and connected to whatever's on the other side. One example is my old motorcycle, which I often say I want to sell but haven't yet because it's part of my past and therefore connected to something deeper. It's a link to another time, and yet it functions in the present, like an old reliable watch. Another example is our black cat Rhonda, named for the first feline Rhonda, who was originally named for the social worker at Fort Lauderdale Hospital. Even though she has her own unique spirit, the cat is a link to the past — a happy reminder of endurance through life's struggles.

And now this book I've written is another thread of constancy from past into present. It gives meaning to the journey. Now it's my responsibility to take this thread forward and weave it into the kind of life I want.

Acknowledgements

M Y deepest gratitude goes to my parents, both of whom remained supportive from the first days of writing and throughout the publication process. My father's encouragement helped motivate me to complete the manuscript, while my mother provided invaluable assistance in the form of memory retrieval. Good memory, it can be said, is both a blessing and a curse, but in the craft of writing it is an exclusive blessing. My mother's impeccable memory is well represented in the early chapters.

Staying with the topic of memory retrieval, I owe a debt of gratitude to the records departments at East Alabama Medical Center, Imperial Point Medical Center and Fort Lauderdale Hospital. Thanks to them, I was able to recover complete copies of my records. These allowed me to recall in detail events that had been previously long forgotten.

Big thanks to friends and family members who offered advice after reading early drafts of the manuscript. These include Phillip Burroughs, Stacey Ballard, Christina Hartman, James Canning, Matthew Keramati and, most especially, Amy

Bluemle. Thank you for muddling through the muck and suggesting improvements that I could not see for myself. I thank my editor, Sue Korbel, for her ability to edit for style, grammar and flow, all with the same eye for quality. I am also thankful to my predecessors in the mental health industry, medicine, and journalism who through their courage to speak out have helped inspire me to do likewise. These include Thomas Szasz, Peter Breggin, Robert Whitaker, Oliver Sacks, Elio Frattaroli and Marcia Angell.

Last, but certainly not least, there is someone who merits special recognition. My wife Sarah deserves a great deal of credit for taking this book forward into the marketplace. If it weren't for her loving support, these words would have remained shelved in our basement as a dusty, unknown manuscript.